SEXUAL DYSFUNCTION IN NEUROLOGICAL DISORDERS

DIAGNOSIS, MANAGEMENT, AND REHABILITATION

Sexual Dysfunction in Neurological Disorders

Diagnosis, Management, and Rehabilitation

François Boller, M.D.
*Associate Professor of
Neurology and Psychiatry
University of Pittsburgh
Pittsburgh, Pennsylvania*

Ellen Frank, Ph.D.
*Assistant Professor of Psychiatry
and Psychology
University of Pittsburgh
Pittsburgh, Pennsylvania*

Foreword by Norman Geschwind, M.D.

Raven Press ■ New York

Raven Press, 1140 Avenue of the Americas, New York, New York 10036

Made in the United States of America

International Standard Book Number 0-89004-500-3
Library of Congress Catalog Number 81-85165

Great care has been taken to maintain the accuracy of the information contained in the volume. However, Raven Press cannot be held responsible for errors or for any consequences arising from the use of the information contained herein.

Materials appearing in this book prepared by individuals as part of their official duties as U.S. Government employees are not covered by the above-mentioned copyright.

Preface

Three years ago, while one of us (F.B.) was responsible for neuroscience teaching to second year medical students at Case Western Reserve University, it was decided to incorporate a lecture on Sexual Dysfunctions in Neurological Disorders into the course. It was quite a surprise to find out that even though several journal articles were addressed to particular aspects of the topic, no comprehensive review was available. Also, while some excellent books on the topic of human sexuality have recently become available, they generally fall short of incorporating material specifically related to neurological disorders. This volume is an expansion of the notes that were put together for that original lecture.

The book reviews the etiology, symptoms, and practical management of impairments of sexual function in patients with neurological disorders. It summarizes the anatomy and physiology of neural structures related to sexual behavior, and reviews the clinical approach to patients with sexual disorders, with emphasis on history-taking and the physical examination.

We have presented nervous system syndromes that produce sexual dysfunctions, with separate sections for diseases of the peripheral nervous system, the spinal cord, and the cerebral hemispheres. We discuss in detail the effects of drugs that interfere with sexual behavior, particularly by direct CNS action. We conclude with a brief review of sexual problems in aging.

We have written the volume in the hope of informing a variety of professionals in health fields, including physicians (particularly neurologists, internists, rehabilitation specialists, and psychiatrists), psychologists, nurses, and allied health personnel involved in rehabilitation. We have made an effort to write in a fashion that makes the book accessible to persons who do not have specific knowledge of the anatomy and physiology of the nervous system, and hope that it will be of value in arresting the long-standing failure of health professionals to address the sexual problems of patients with neurological disorders.

F.B.
E.F.
Pittsburgh, August 1981

Contents

Acknowledgments

Many of our colleagues helped us put this volume together. We are particularly indebted to Otto Appenzeller, M.D., D. Frank Benson, M.D., Monroe Cole, M.D., Michael Eisenberg, Ph.D., Joseph M. Foley, M.D., Muriel Lezak, Ph.D., and Oscar M. Reinmuth, M.D., who provided very useful and constructive comments on early versions of the manuscript.

Very valuable technical help was received from Ms. Barbara Good, Ms. Carol Gore, and Ms. Mary Whalen. Ms. Mag Maloney from the Media Production Services of Western Psychiatric Institute and Clinic skillfully drew some of the illustrations. We also wish to acknowledge our debt to the staff of Raven Press and particularly to Dr. Diana M. Schneider, Executive Editor, and Ms. Rita Scheman, Assistant Managing Editor, whose patient contributions guided us through the final steps of the preparation of the book.

Finally we want to thank Norman Geschwind, M.D., for kindly accepting to write the Foreword to this book.

Research was supported in part by the Medical Research Service of the Veterans Administration and by Western Psychiatric Institute and Clinic.

Foreword

François Boller and Ellen Frank point out in their introductory chapter to this volume that despite the great freedom in the discussion of sexual issues that has characterized both the recent history of medicine and society in general, there has been a remarkable lack of interest in the issues of sexual dysfunctions related to neurological disease. Although there have been detailed discussions of the sexual problems of patients with spinal injuries or with temporal lobe epilepsy in specialized publications, there is probably no overview of this important field. It is easy to be aware of the general neglect of this subject. It has been my experience that even in histories taken by psychiatric residents of patients with behavioral changes in temporal lobe epilepsy, there is often a failure to obtain a detailed account of the frequently dramatic alterations in sexual activities. This monograph provides an easily readable, short summary of most types of sexual dysfunction that occur with lesions at all levels of the nervous system and provides a useful guide to diagnosis and management.

It is worth pointing out that the study of relationships between sexuality and the brain is only in its infancy. Before World War II, most such discussions centered on the alterations in sexual behavior that occurred from lesions of peripheral nerve or spinal cord. More recently, there has been increasing interest in the sexual changes that occur with lesions at higher levels and with alterations of sexuality in epilepsy. Many investigations in the last quarter-century have revealed much new information concerning the relationships between sex and the nervous system, and this body of data, although not generally well known, will undoubtedly produce a revolution in our thinking in years to come.

A Darwinian viewpoint leads to the obvious conclusion that in the final analysis, survival of the fittest means success in reproduction. It is therefore not surprising that in the course of evolution, the nervous system and other organs have developed important mechanisms to serve this end. Indeed, sexual differentiation is present in the very warp and woof of the body in general and the nervous system in particular. Every cell in the body contains sexual marking in its chromosomes that are either XX or XY. Even more remarkable, however, is the extent to which many organs and parts of the body that at first glance do not appear to be directly involved in sexual behavior are characterized by the presence of specialized accumulations of either androgens or estrogens, or, in some cases, probably both. Motor nerves and skeletal muscle accumulate androgens, which of course explains the fact that female athletes sometimes use testosterone to increase muscular development. At nearly all levels of the nervous system, there are cells that accumulate either androgens or estrogens, or both hormones. Among songbirds it is the male who sings, and Nottebohm and colleagues (Nottebohn and Arnold, 1976; and Nottebohn, 1976) have shown that the region of the central nervous system involved in song is functionally lateralized to one side of the brain and contains testosterone receptors. Castration abolishes song. On the other hand, if the young female is exposed to testosterone, she too sings. Raisman and Field (1971) have shown that there is a region in the brain of the rat whose cellular structure differs according to the sex of the animal. It has also been shown that early exposure of the female to testosterone induces a similar change in structure. The presence of androgens in early life is necessary for masculine differentiation of the brain. On the other hand, exposure of female rats in early life to androgens induces persistent alterations in adult behavior, both sexual and nonsexual. It has been shown recently that all, or nearly all, norepinephrine-containing neurons in the central nervous system of rodents accumulate estrogens. Many brain cells have the capacity to synthesize estrogens from the appropriate precursors.

There are many disorders that are sexually differentiated. In nearly all the developmental disorders of language, learning, and behavior in childhood males predominate with the result that institutions for learning disabilities and pediatric mental hospitals have predominantly male populations. These conditions include dyslexia, stuttering, autism, hyperactivity, and delayed speech. In later childhood and adolescence, there is a male predominance in the Tourette syndrome, the Kleine-Levin syndrome, and delinquency, while females predominate in anorexia nervosa and hysteria. Although in some of these conditions there may be important cultural and personal environmental factors, it is still likely that these are occurring on a background of biological predisposition.

In later life there are again disorders that are separated sexually. Autoimmune diseases such as myasthenia gravis, lupus erythematosus, and probably multiple sclerosis predominate in women, while others such as amyotrophic lateral sclerosis predominate in men.

It seems likely that in the next 25 years there will be an increasingly rapid growth in knowledge about the hormonal effects on the nervous system and about sexual differentiation, as well as a more penetrating insight into the pathogenesis of disorders which differentially affect males and females. Simultaneously, there will certainly be increasing awareness of the many ways in which damage, excessive stimulation, or drugs acting on the nervous system may produce alterations in sexual behavior. The combination of the two bodies of knowledge should undoubtedly lead to new and powerful therapeutic methods. I hope that those who read this excellent summary by François Boller and Ellen Frank of current knowledge of the effects of damage to the nervous system will have their appetites whetted to look further into the ever-growing literature and to participate in the new advances of knowledge in the field of sexuality as related to the brain.

Norman   Geschwind, M.D.
James Jackson Putnam Professor of Neurology
Harvard Medical School

Professor of Psychology
Massachusetts Institute of Technology

Director, Neurological Unit
Beth Israel Hospital

Boston, February 25, 1981

Chapter 1

Introduction

Disorders of sexual function occur frequently in patients with neurological disease but, with few exceptions, have been sorely neglected in the literature. The frequent occurrence of these disorders is clearly related to the fact that the sexual organs are directly controlled by components at all levels of the nervous system, ranging from the peripheral nerves to the cerebral hemispheres. In addition, it must be emphasized that sexuality is not just a biological function but also has complex psychological and social aspects. The work of ethologists such as Konrad Lorenz (1970) has shown this to be true for most animal species. In humans, however, these aspects of sexuality appear particularly preponderant. Frequently, how well individuals perform sexually determines how much of a "man" (or a "woman") they see themselves to be and, in turn, may determine how adequate a person they believe themselves to be. Given this system of belief with respect to the emphasis on sexuality and sexual performance, a great deal of anxiety becomes attached to situations in which sexual behavior is expected. These added meanings and expectations have added considerable importance to sexual behavior and have contributed to the fact that human sexuality consists of much more than a reproductive function. These factors may help explain why sexual functions are highly vulnerable to all types of severe and chronic diseases, and particularly to diseases of the nervous system, which so frequently disrupt motor and cognitive behavior.

The scarcity of published material on this topic is therefore difficult to explain. Supposedly, the subject of sex is no longer taboo, yet physicians and other health care professionals all too often neglect the subject of sexual functioning with their patients; patients, in turn, often hesitate to volunteer symptoms related to what is considered, rightly or wrongly, a highly private part of their lives. Changes are occurring, however. In a recent bibliographical review of the literature on the general topic of sex and disability, Eisenberg (1978) notes that of the 925 papers he found on the subject, over 80% were published after 1960. New journals devoted to the relationship between medical problems and sexuality, such as *Medical Aspects of Human Sexuality* and the recently founded *Sexuality and Disability*, do publish a few articles on the subject of sex and neurological disorders. The lack of articles relating sexual disorders to neurological diseases has one notable exception, spinal cord injuries (for which Eisenberg lists 135 references) and, to a lesser extent, such specific conditions as epilepsy (Blumer and Walker, 1975) and diabetes (Ellenberg, 1971; Karacan et al., 1978).

Despite the increased awareness of the importance of sexuality at the research and publication level, in the past, medical school curriculae and other training programs for health professionals have failed to provide adequate education in the area of human sexuality, and most care givers remain poorly prepared to diagnose and treat sexual problems. Furthermore, because of their general ignorance in this area, most health care professionals are reluctant to initiate a discussion of sexual problems with patients.

This volume will review the etiology, symptoms, and practical management of sexual dysfunction in patients with neurological disorders. We shall first summarize the anatomy and physiology of neural structures related to sexual behavior and then review the clinical approach to patients with sexual disorders with emphasis on history-taking and on physical examination.

The description of CNS syndromes that produce sexual dysfunction will begin with a review of diseases of the peripheral nervous system, particularly peripheral neuropathies. We shall then review spinal cord injuries and other lesions of the spinal cord that affect sexual function; this is probably the area in which the largest amount of information is currently available in the literature. Next, we will deal with lesions of the cerebral hemispheres, including lesions that do not directly affect the function of genital organs but interfere with sexuality because of their impact on motor, affective, or cognitive behavior. This class of disorders has received particularly scant attention. We shall next discuss in detail drugs that interfere with sexual behavior, particularly those that do so by direct CNS action. Finally, we shall review some of the literature on sexual behavior in the aging.

Important distinctions must be made in the discussion of sexual difficulties. Loss or decrease of libido refers to an impairment of sexual drive and sexual urge; impotence is defined as a disturbance of sexual function in the male that precludes satisfactory coitus (Masters and Johnson, 1966). It is generally agreed, however, that a patient who has satisfactory penile rigidity and who is able to engage in coitus but who is unable to achieve an orgasm or to ejaculate is not, in the strictest sense, impotent (Furlow, 1979). In the male, it may be useful to further distinguish between primary impotence (i.e., cases in which sexual functioning has never developed normally) and secondary impotence (sexual difficulties that arise in postpubertal life, following a history of effective sexual functioning). In this volume, we shall deal principally with the problem of secondary impotence and disorders that are acquired after puberty. There is no corresponding term for impotence in the female, where the term frigidity has been loosely applied to several types of sexual disorders.

Recently, sexual disorders in the female have been divided into three general categories: 1) inhibition of desire, which is essentially the same as loss or decrease of libido, 2) arousal phase disorders in which the female fails to lubricate vaginally and/or fails to achieve psychological arousal, and 3) anorgasmia in which arousal takes place, but orgasm is not achieved. As in the male, these difficulties can be either primary or secondary in origin. Finally, sterility in males, refers to the inability to emit viable, mobile spermatozoa; in females, it refers to the inability to conceive and bear children.

As will be seen throughout this volume, there has been very little research describing or attempting to explain the effects of neurological disorders on the sexual behavior of females. The causes for the paucity of information on this topic and on female sexual dysfunction in general are quite complex and often far from clear. It is generally agreed that these causes include a double standard with respect to sexuality: It is assumed that sexual function is of greater importance to men than to women; that sexual problems of females are less apparent, both to their partners and to themselves, than are the sexual problems of males; that for the most part, exploration of sexual problems in the female requires that a female patient respond to questions from a male physician although it is usually considerably easier to discuss such problems with someone of the same sex; and finally, that there exists a general tendency in all medical research to concentrate on male patients as opposed to female patients. Further discussion of this particular aspect of the problem will be found in the chapters illustrating the various clinical syndromes.

In recent years, considerable advances have been made in the management of sexual dysfunctions. This certainly applies also to sexual disorders of neurological origin including those that are secondary to irreversible neurological diseases such as severe spinal cord traumas. In all the cases in which suitable information is available, we shall outline in some detail the appropriate principles of practical management and therapy.

To conclude this introduction, we would like to discuss some general factors which are essential for the recognition and treatment of sexual disorders of neurological origin. It is clearly necessary for all physicians and allied health care professionals to have an appropriate background and knowledge of the anatomical, physiological, and psychological basis of human sexuality. They should make a point to routinely explore possible sexual problems with virtually all patients. How often does this occur at the present time? Pinderhughes and co-workers (1972), investigated the extent to which physicians and patients discuss sex-related matters; they used two questionnaires, one presented to the medical staff (resident physicians, staff physicians, and consultants) and one to patients of the VA Hospital in Boston. Physicians reported that they initiated discussion of sexual matters in about 40% of cases. Interestingly, patients reported an even lower rate of doctor-initiated discussion (25%). Both doctors and patients agreed that few patients (about 20%) initiate discussion on sex-related problems. It can only be assumed that rates in a general hospital, which would include both female and male patients, would be even lower than those reported by Pinderhughes and co-workers. The reasons for these low percentages are certainly complex, but they clearly indicate that the present level of doctor–patient communication on sex problems is far from satisfactory. No precise data exist at the present time about the extent of communication on sex problems between patients and health personnel other than physicians, but some data suggest that it is somehow greater than that between patients and physicians. These data will be discussed later in this volume (page 57).

Sexual dysfunction frequently accompanies a variety of neurological disorders. When confronted by patients with known neurological diseases who complain of sexual difficulties, one often faces a problem of differential diagnosis. First, it is important to remember that the base rates of these problems in the physically healthy general population are far from zero. For example, in a study of 100 nonpatient couples, Frank and co-workers (1978), found that nearly one-half of the women experienced difficulty with orgasm, approximately 17% of the men experienced erectile problems, and fully one-third of the men reported premature ejaculation. It is also necessary to keep in mind that clinical studies show that in the overall population a large number of sexual disorders in both females and males are related to "psychological" factors (Simpson, 1950; Masters and Johnson, 1970; Cooper, 1972; Levine, 1976; Small, 1978). Other causes of sexual dysfunction include endocrine disorders, medical diseases, and genitourinary problems (especially those associated with surgery). It is often said (e.g., Weiss, 1972) that endocrine disorders involving sexual dysfunction are characterized by decreased or absent libido. This rule of thumb may be true in many cases, but, as we shall see, some neurological disorders such as temporal lobe epilepsy may also impair libido without demonstrable endocrine abnormalities. The diagnosis of psychogenic causes of sexual problems must be kept in mind, especially when such problems are episodic. This, of course, is more difficult to document in females than in males in whom nocturnal erections can be recorded either by history or objectively (Karacan et al., 1966; Fisher et al., 1975; Jovanovic, 1967; Wasserman et al., 1980). However, the opposite may also occur; some of the sexual problems we shall discuss may actually be the presenting signs in conditions such as diabetes, multiple sclerosis, or amyloidosis. In this case there is the possibility of mistakenly considering as psychological a problem that is not. Abel (*personal communication*, 1980) argues that 66% of male sexual problems can be correctly categorized as either organic or psychogenic by asking these five questions: Was the onset of the problem slow, that is, requiring more than one month or rapid, that is, requiring less than one month? Is the occurrence of the problem continuous or intermittent? Is the problem present during nonintercourse-related sex, that is, masturbation and other forms of sexual contact? Are morning erections present? Does sexual interest or drive remain? Abel associates slow onset, continuous occurrence, presence of the problem during nonintercourse-related sex, and sustained sexual drive with organic etiology. Rapid onset, intermittent occurrence, absence of the problem during masturbation and lack of sustained drive suggest instead a psychogenic etiology. A differential diagnosis is of course easier when sexual problems appear in a context of a clear neurological disorder. Here again one must remember, however, that, as pointed out by Griffith and Trieschmann (1975), most organic (or, in their terminology, "primary") sexual dysfunctions entail a psychological (or "secondary") component, which must be kept in mind for purpose of proper diagnosis, prognosis, and treatment.

In most instances, diagnosis and therapy of sexual disorders logically rests on the primary physician. It would be just as logical and also convenient if physicians could avail themselves of the cooperation of persons specialized in the field of sexual disorders. At the present time, however, these persons are few. In addition, many sex therapists at present screen their patients and tend to eliminate anyone with an organic disorder. As a consequence, many have little or no experience in the special field of sexual dysfunction associated with neurological diseases. The example of some spinal cord injury units that have organized special multidisciplinary teams (Eisenberg and Rastad, 1976) should be followed to a much wider extent. The formation of such teams could produce some of the knowledge that is at present strikingly absent in many areas and could lead to improved treatment of sexual disorders. Finally, in many instances the patient can be greatly assisted by his or her participation in self-help groups made up of other patients. In many instances, patients with specific injuries who have been able to overcome all or part of the sexual problems they have experienced can be of great help to other patients experiencing similar difficulties. First, it is frequently easier for the distressed patients to explain and discuss their problem with someone who has a comparable disability. Second, within these self-help groups the leaders often have more experience in explaining how sexual problems can be overcome than do health care professionals.

Chapter 2

Anatomy and Physiology

Most of our knowledge of the anatomy and physiology of the neurological structures responsible for sexual functions relates to the periphery. This includes the lower segments of the spinal cord and their connections with the sexual orgasm via the nerve roots and the peripheral nerves (see Johnson and Spalding, 1974, and Appenzeller, 1976 for recent reviews). Blumer and Walker (1975) have recently reviewed a number of studies concerning the areas of the cortex related to sexuality. Almost nothing is known about the centers and pathways between the cortex and the spinal cord.

AUTONOMIC AND PERIPHERAL INNERVATION

The autonomic nervous system (ANS) is responsible for the greatest part of the innervation of the sexual organs, as well as many other organs and systems such as the eyes, many glands, much of the gastrointestinal system, the cardiovascular system, etc. It is so named in contrast to the somatic or voluntary nervous system that innervates, for example, voluntary muscles and transmits sensation from the skin.

The ANS nerve fibers that reach the organs with autonomic innervation originate from autonomic ganglion cells and are therefore called postganglionic. In turn, the ganglion cells are activated by preganglionic nerve fibers that originate in the spinal cord and in the brain stem.

A brief outline of the anatomy of the spinal cord may help the reader to better understand the organization of the ANS. The spinal cord (Fig. 1) is customarily subdivided into various portions called, from top to bottom, the cervical, the thoracic, the lumbar, and the sacral portion with an additional coccygeal portion of little functional importance. In turn, each portion is divided into several segments that are identified

9

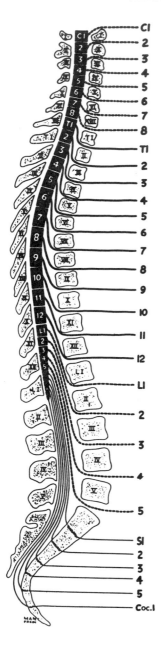

FIG. 1. Schematic drawing of the spinal cord segments and their relationship with the spinal canal and the vertebral bodies. (Reproduced by permission from Haymaker W, Woodhall B: *Peripheral Nerve Injuries: Principles of Diagnosis.* Philadelphia: Saunders, 1953.)

with a letter and a number corresponding to the portion in which they are found. There are eight cervical segments (C_1 to C_8), 12 thoracic segments (T_1 to T_{12}), five lumbar segments (L_1 to L_5), five sacral segments (S_1 to S_5), and one coccygeal segment (Co_1). Each segment has a pair of nerve roots (spinal nerves): the anterior root contains motor fibers, and the posterior root contains sensory fibers, with the exception of the first cervical and the coccygeal segment, that usually contain no posterior roots. Up to the third month of fetal life, the spinal cord occupies the entire length of the vertebral canal, but after that time the rate of growth of the vertebral canal becomes greater than that of the cord, and, in the adult, the spinal cord terminates between the first and second lumbar vertebra. The site of emergence of the spinal nerves does not change and, therefore, the roots have a descending course before exiting from the spinal canal. In the lower part of the canal these roots form the so-called cauda equina. After exiting from the canal the spinal nerves go to the periphery directly, sometimes after forming a network known as plexus.

The ANS is classically subdivided into sympathetic and parasympathetic components. The sympathetic ganglion cells tend to be located in the sympathetic chain, a series of ganglionic cells that are located fairly close to the spinal cord. Their preganglionic fibers originate in the thoracic and lumbar segments of the spinal cord and tend to be short, while their postganglionic fibers tend to be long. The reverse is true for the parasympathetic nerve cells that tend to be located in close proximity to the organs they innervate. Their preganglionic fibers tend to be long and originate either in the brain stem or in the most caudal part of the spinal cord. Perhaps more importantly, stimulation of the sympathetic ganglion cells or of their postganglionic fibers often (but not always) produces the release of noradrenaline (or norepinephrine), whereas parasympathetic ganglion cells or postganglionic fibers tend to release acetylcholine. On this basis it has been proposed to replace the terms sympathetic and parasympathetic and to use instead the more functionally oriented terms of adrenergic and cholinergic systems. However, as is often the case, the older terminology also continues to remain in use.

In addition to fibers that go from the center to the periphery (efferent fibers), the ANS includes fibers connecting the periphery with the central nervous system (CNS) (afferent fibers). They carry sensory impulses from the peripheral organs they innervate to the CNS.

The sympathetic and parasympathetic components of the ANS were originally considered to have opposite and mutually exclusive functions, i.e., to be antagonists. Although this may be partially true for certain organs (e.g., parts of the digestive system), the innervation of the genital system provides a good example of interaction between the two traditional components of the ANS (sympathetic and parasympathetic) and the somatic nervous system as well.

In the male (Figs. 2 and 3; Table 1A), the sympathetic nervous system supplies fibers to the vas deferens, seminal vesicles, the prostate, and the testes (Sjöstrand, 1965). The cells of origin of the preganglionic

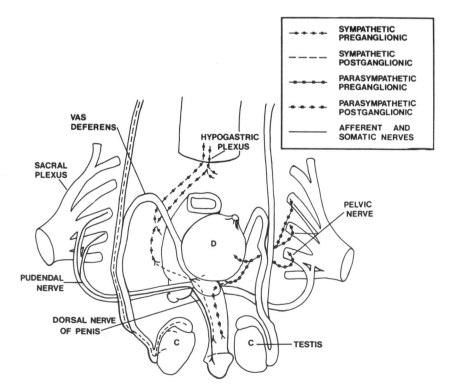

FIG. 2. Schematic drawing of the nerve supply to the male sexual organs. C = testis; D = urinary bladder.

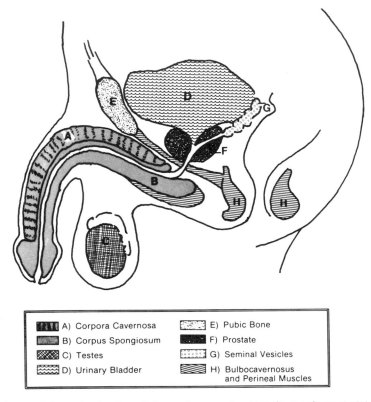

FIG. 3. Schematic drawing of the male sexual organs in a quiescent state.

TABLE 1A. *Innervation of sexual organs: males*

Origin	Action
Parasympathetic-pelvic nerves *nervi erigentes* S_2 to S_4	Reflexogenic erection (?)
Sympathetic-hypogastric nerves T_{10} to L_2	"Psychogenic" erection (?)
	Semen emission
Somatic-pudendal nerves S_2 to S_4	Ejaculation

fibers form a distinct group in the gray matter of the cord known as the intermediolateral column (Fig. 4). The sympathetic fibers innervating sexual organs are in the intermediolateral columns of the lower thoracic (T_{10} to T_{12}) and upper lumbar (L_1 to L_2) segments of the spinal cord. These preganglionic fibers follow the presacral and hypogastric nerves (Fig. 2). They end for the most part in the hypogastric plexus or close to the structures they supply. The postganglionic fibers with which they synapse form a plexus in the proximity of the smooth muscles of the end-organs. From these same organs comes an afferent (sensory) sympathetic system that follows in reverse the course of the sympathetic efferents and enters the spinal cord at the lower thoracic and upper lumbar (T_{10} to L_1) level.

The preganglionic parasympathetic fibers originate in the intermediolateral nucleus of the sacral (S_2 to S_4) spinal cord. The fibers travel in the S_2 to S_4 ventral roots and form the pelvic nerves. Classical

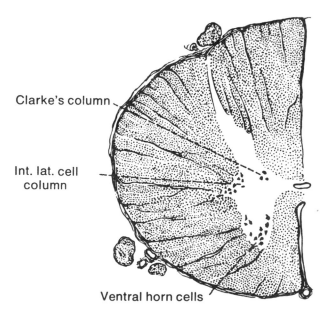

Clarke's column

Int. lat. cell column

Ventral horn cells

FIG. 4. Section of the spinal cord at the midthoracic level. The intermediolateral wall column contains the cells of origin of the sympathetic preganglionic fibers. (Reproduced by permission from Brodal A: *Neurological Anatomy*. London: Oxford University Press, 1981.)

anatomists, who noticed that their stimulation tended to induce erection in experimental animals, named the pelvic nerves *nervi erigentes*. These fibers join the hypogastric plexus and end in the erectile tissue of the corpora cavernosa and corpus spongiosum of the penis. Parasympathetic fibers also reach the prostate, seminal vesicles, vas deferens, and the ejaculatory ducts. An afferent parasympathetic system follows the same course entering the spinal cord at the posterior roots of S_2 to S_4.

The somatic (voluntary) innervation originates from the anterior horn cells of S_2 to S_4. These fibers travel in the pudendal nerves (Fig. 5) and end in the bulbocavernosus and ischiocavernosus muscles. The pudendal nerves also carry sensory fibers responsible for skin sensation over the S_2 to S_5 dermatomes. This includes the so-called saddle area surrounding and including the anus, the scrotum, and the penis.

As stated above, the sequence of neurological events involved in sexual function in the male requires harmonious participation of the parasympathetic, sympathetic, and somatic divisions of the nervous system. Erection occurs as a result of vasocongestion within the sponge-like erectile tissue of the corpora cavernosa and corpus spongiosum of the penis. Stimulation of the pelvic (parasympathetic) nerves produces dilation of the arteries and constriction of the veins of these spongy tissues, thus causing and maintaining erection (Weiss, 1972). Although most authors agree that the action of the parasympathetic nervous system is primarily responsible for erection, it is probable that sympathetic activity can also produce it (Bors and Turner, 1967). This conclusion is based in part on the fact that erection is found even in patients with documented lesions at several different levels of the spinal cord including the sacral spinal cord (Kahn, 1950; Comarr, 1970). It has been postulated that the sacral (parasympathetic) erection center is primarily responsible for reflexogenic erection; i.e., erection produced by direct physical stimulation of the genitals, whereas the thoracolumbar (sympathetic) erection center mediates psychogenic erection produced by mental stimuli. Ordinarily both centers act synergistically to produce penile erection (Weiss, 1972).

The neurological events leading to ejaculation are more complex than those of erection. In order for semen to be emitted, it must first be expelled into the prostatic urethra, a process that is dependent on the

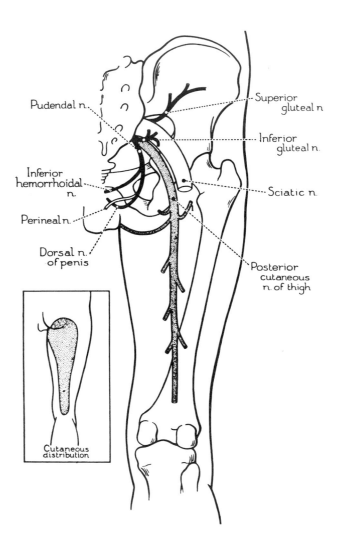

FIG. 5. Pudendal nerve after its origin from the sacral plexus and its exit into the ischiorectal fossa. The dorsal nerve of the penis contains both motor and sensory fibers, but in the female, this branch (called dorsal nerve of the clitoris) only carries afferent (sensory) fibers. (Reproduced by permission from Haymaker W, Woodhall B: *Peripheral Nerve Injuries: Principles of Diagnosis*. Philadelphia: Saunders, 1953.)

hypogastric sympathetic nerves. Emission and ejaculation are caused by contraction of the bulbocavernosus and ischiocavernosus muscles mediated by the pudendal (somatic) nerves.

In the female (Figs. 6 and 7; Table 1B), the ovaries are innervated mainly by the sympathetic nervous system. The preganglionic fibers originate in the intermediolateral column at the lower thoracic (T_{10} to T_{11}) level and are part of the splanchnic nerves up to their synapses in the ovarian ganglion located near the origin of the ovarian artery. The postganglionic fibers constitute the ovarian plexus. This is a continuation of the aortic and renal plexus and follows the course of the ovarian artery and vein and supplies fibers to the ovary. It also supplies the Fallopian tubes and the broad ligament, which receive additional sympathetic supply from the hypogastric plexus and parasympathetic supply from the uterine plexus. This pattern of mixed sympathetic and parasympathetic supply applies also to the uterus (although it is not universally agreed that the uterus receives any parasympathetic supply) and to the vagina. As in the male, the parasympathetic supply derives from the S_2 to S_4 sacral segments and follows the pelvic nerves.

The somatic nervous supply to the female genital organs is provided by the pudendal nerve (Fig. 5), which, as in the male, arises from the S_2 to S_4 segments of the spinal cord and passes to the lateral wall of the ischiorectal fossa, where it gives off the interior hemorrhoidal nerve and then divides into two terminal branches. The first is the perineal nerve that supplies sensory fibers to the vulva and motor fibers to the superficial perineal muscles, the anal and vaginal sphincters, and levatores ani. The other terminal branch is the dorsal nerve of the clitoris which is purely afferent (sensory). Its sensory receptors are located in relation to the cavernous tissue, which receives efferent (vasomotor) innervation from parasympathetic fibers to the cavernous plexus.

The role of the ANS in the physiology of female sexual organs, particularly the ovaries, the tubes, and the uterus is not entirely clear, but most authors agree that it is not essential as far as fertility is concerned (Brodal, 1981), since females with a denervated uterus can menstruate, become pregnant, and deliver normally, as has been observed in experimental animals and in women with neurological lesions. The role of the neural supply to the clitoris and other parts of the

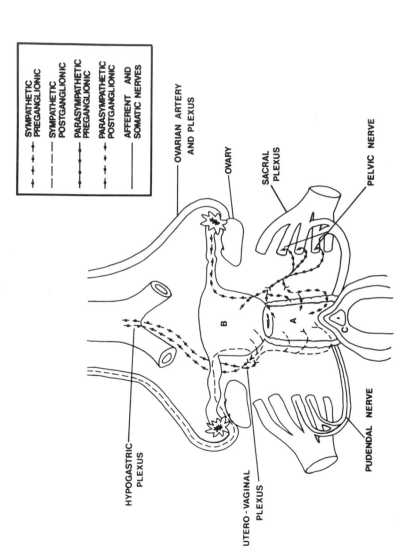

FIG. 6. Schematic drawing of the nerve supply to the female sexual organs.
A = vagina; B = uterus; C = clitoris.

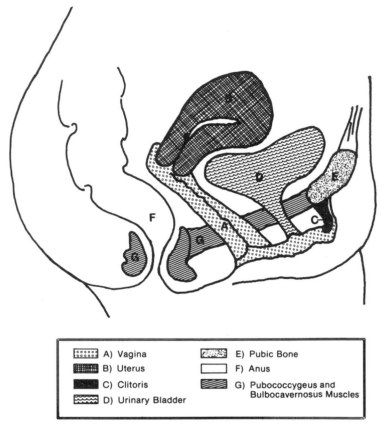

FIG. 7. Schematic drawing of the female sexual organs in quiescent state.

external genitals is certainly much greater. The parasympathetic nervous system contributes to the microscopic and, when present, macroscopic intumescence (swelling) of the clitoris and produces increased vaginal secretion. Intumescence of the clitoris has been thought of as the equivalent of erection in the male; it must be noted, however, that the clitoris is a unique organ limited in its physiologic function to initiating and elevating levels of sexual tension. No such organ exists in the male (Masters and Johnson, 1966). It is also obvious that there is no event in the sexual function of females that is a true counterpart of the male ejaculation. Here again, however, some authors consider contraction

TABLE 1B. *Innervation of sexual organs: Females*

Origin	Action
Parasympathetic-pelvic nerves S_2 to S_4	Intumescence of clitoris; vaginal secretion
Sympathetic-splanchnic nerves ovarian plexus T_{10} to L_2	Contraction of smooth muscles of tubes and uterus
Somatic-pudendal nerves S_2 to S_4	Contraction of vaginal sphincter and pelvic floor

of the smooth muscles of the uterine tubes and uterus (under sympathetic control) equivalent to emission in males, while the rhythmic contractions of the bulbospongiosus (vaginal sphincter) and ischiocavernosus muscles and of the pelvic floor (under somatic nerve control) have been compared to ejaculation (Tarabulcy, 1972). Although it is true that these events are mediated by the same nervous supply (Tables 1A and 1B) and occur in a corresponding phase of the orgasmic cycle in both sexes, this comparison appears arbitrary and may be misleading. The loss of emission and ejaculation in the male seems in fact to have different physiological and psychological consequences than a loss of corresponding events in the female.

As noted in a recent study (Graber and Kline-Graber, 1979), female orgasm may be compared to a reflex loop containing basically two components, a sensory or afferent loop and a motor or efferent loop. These authors have shown that contraction of circumvaginal muscles (the pubococcygeus muscles) is impaired in women who fail to achieve orgasm. Their conclusion is that the pubococcygeus muscle plays an important part in the pathophysiology of female orgasm even though it is not clear whether this is important at the level of the afferent side of the reflex loop, efferent side, or both.

SPINAL CORD PATHWAYS, BRAIN STEM, AND THALAMUS

The previous section has dealt with the current knowledge of the anatomical structures of the spinal cord thought to be responsible for the innervation of sexual organs. The connections between these areas and the higher segments of the CNS are far from clear. Our limited knowledge of the spinal cord localization of pathways related to sexual behavior derives essentially from neurosurgical material. Partial cordotomies undertaken for the treatment of intractable pain suggest that the sexual pathways are located in the anterolateral column of the spinal cord and in the lateral portion of the medulla, presumably in close association with the spinothalamic pathways (Olivecrona, 1947). It is not known whether this association continues in the pons, mesencephalon, and thalamus. Blumer and Walker (1975) noticed the remarkable absence of reports of genital responses in the abundant literature on stereotaxic thalamic stimulations and lesions. The only exceptions appear to be the reports by MacLean (1973) that stimulation of parts of the thalamus at times produces erection and ejaculation in the squirrel monkey (Saimiri sciureus) (see below).

HYPOTHALAMUS

Lisk (1967) summarized well the role of specific parts of the hypothalamus in sexual behavior in various animal species. A hypothalamic center located in the preoptic area appears to be responsible for the initiation of copulation. Implants of hormones (estrogen or testosterone propionate) and electrical stimulation of this area elicit a copulatory response, whereas lesions decrease sexual behavior. Hormonal treatment does not reverse this change. A second center, located in the median eminence area, regulates gonadotropin release. Mating ability decreases in animals following lesions of this area but can be restored by hormonal replacement.

Human studies vary in the importance attributed to the hypothalamus (and to hormones in general) in sexual behavior. In both males and females, appropriate increases in the levels of androgenic and, respectively, estrogenic hormones are necessary for puberty to occur. In males, once normal sexual function is established, a severe androgenic deficiency must be present before sexuality is seriously impaired, and the onset of impotence and loss of libido lag behind the loss of androgenic function. Martin and co-workers (1977) recently reviewed in detail the relationship between sex hormones and sexual functions.

Bauer (1959) has summarized the clinical findings of 60 patients with autopsy-proven hypothalamic pathology. Nearly one-half of the patients (28 cases) had hypogonadism associated with dysthermia. Pathology in these cases tended to involve the anterior hypothalamus. Twenty-four of the cases (19 males and 5 females) had precocious puberty. Only few of these patients had eye signs and diabetes insipidus. On this basis, Bauer expressed the belief that precocious puberty was associated particularly with lesions of the posterior hypothalamus. It is noteworthy that none of his patients exhibited hypersexuality.

CEREBRAL HEMISPHERES

In the classical Klüver-Bucy syndrome (1939), male rhesus monkeys with bilateral temporal lobectomy exhibited a series of striking behavior changes. These animals, which prior to the operation were wild and aggressive, became tame and placid after surgery. Other changes included visual agnosia (psychic blindness), strong oral tendencies, and hypermetamorphosis (irresistible impulse to act). The animals also had changes in sexual behavior. In the authors' words, the monkeys appeared "hypersexed"; this was evident when they were alone (spontaneous erections), with a human observer ("presenting reactions" on approach of an observer), or with other monkeys, at which time various forms of heterosexual and homosexual behavior could be observed. Some authors (see Appenzeller, 1976, p. 289 for a review) have questioned whether this behavior represents true hypersexuality. Nevertheless, there is no question that the Klüver-Bucy syndrome represents a milestone in the study of the relationship between the temporal lobes and sexual functions. Hypersexual behavior has also been claimed in the monkey and in the cat following lesions of the amygdala and overlying piriform cortex or small lesions of the piriform cortex (Green et al., 1957; Orback et al., 1960). In animals the effect of cerebral lesions varies with sex; removal of the entire neocortex does not interfere with the maintenance of mating behavior in either the female cat or the female rat (Bard, 1939). In male rats, however, Beach (1940) found that a destruction of more than 20% of the cortex interfered with copulatory behavior, and that no rat with more than 59% damage was able to copulate. Testosterone proprionate did not reverse this change.

As briefly mentioned earlier, MacLean and colleagues (MacLean and Ploog, 1962; MacLean et al., 1963; MacLean, 1973; Dua and Mac-Lean, 1964) described several brain areas where electrical stimulation produced penile erection in the squirrel monkey. Such areas were found in the medulla, pons, midbrain, septal area, hypothalamus, medial forebrain bundle, anterior thalamus, and medial frontal cortex. Seminal discharge occurred only when stimulation was applied along the course of the spinothalamic pathway and its projections into the intralaminal region of the thalamus (MacLean et al., 1963). However, three facts must be kept in mind in considering these results. Erection in the squirrel monkey is frequently used for purposes not directly related to sexual activity, e.g., greeting and dominance display; these experiments were all carried out on monkeys immobilized in a monkey chair, so that it is not possible to determine whether stimulation would have produced any change in behavior toward female squirrel monkeys. Finally, analogous experiments in the female elicited no sexual response whatsoever.

Robinson and Mishkin (1968) studied penile erection in *Macaca mulatta* and also found many areas from which erection could be obtained. They noted, however, that in an unrestrained situation, males with stimulated erection and females actually only copulated "in a minority of instances." As can be seen, it is not entirely clear that these responses represent true sexual arousal.

Cortical areas related to sexual behavior in humans will be discussed in a later section of this volume (pp. 50–61).

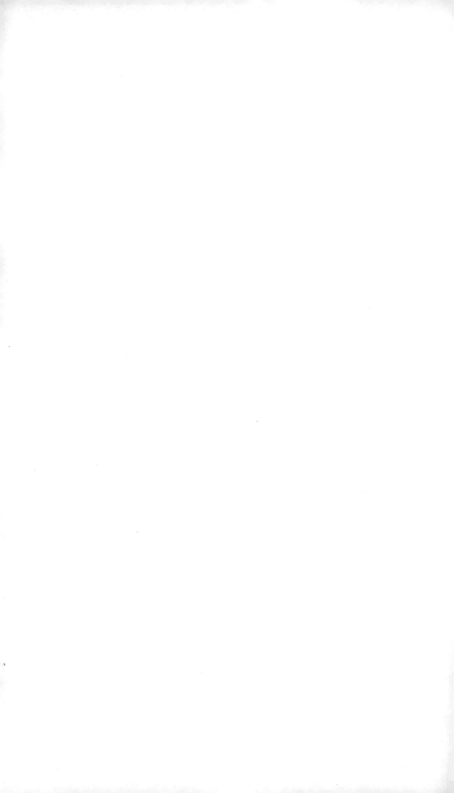

Chapter 3

Approach to the Patient with Sexual Problems

As is the case with all clinical problems, the most important step in the diagnosis and therapy of patients with sexual difficulties consists of a detailed history and physical examination. In a hospital or at the doctor's office, the patient with diseases of the nervous system will, on occasion, volunteer a sexual problem as a chief complaint and/or as reason for referral, either as an isolated problem or among other symptoms. Much more frequently, however, the patient will report sexual inadequacies only on direct questioning. Questions about sexual behavior should therefore be a routine part of history taking in every patient. Some patients will respond candidly, whereas others will be reluctant to discuss the subject. We believe that when questions are asked without evidence of prejudice or preconceived ideas, and that once patients understand that such inquiry is used only to gain a better understanding of their problems, few, if any, will refuse to answer and will be offended.

The form and content of history taking must, of course, be placed in the context of the psychological and social conditions of the individual patient. Furthermore, the patient's comfort in discussing what are generally regarded as highly personal aspects of life can be greatly enhanced if the examiner follows a few simple guidelines. First, examiners themselves must be as comfortable as possible with this line of inquiry. The clinician who finds that he or she experiences some discomfort or anxiety when questioning patients about sexuality should either engage in a self-desensitization process (taking a sexual history from a few friends and asking the questions to a mirror may both be effective techniques) or take a brief professional development course in the assessment and treatment of sexual problems. A second important step in helping patients to feel more comfortable is to give patients permission to use *any* terminology they know from the anatomical names to street language to describe how they are functioning. Third, it is often useful, having made this request, to promise patients that you, the examiner, will stop them if you do not understand their terminology, if they will promise to stop you when they do not understand yours.

Once the clinician senses that the patient has been made as comfortable as possible, the current level of sexual drive and sexual performance must be determined and recorded; but just as importantly, the examiner must establish whether the present level of performance represents a change. Specifically, the examiner should inquire about sexual drive and desire; occurrence of erection under various circumstances, including nocturnal erections in the male; nature and role of sexual fantasies; and masturbation, distinguishing between simple manipulation of sexual organs and actual orgasm-directed self-stimulation. The frequency and timing of such events should be determined by direct questioning, which should take the form, "How often do you..." or "How frequently do you...", since this form of questioning is much more likely to produce an accurate picture of the patient's functioning than the form, "Do you ever...". In the area of sexuality, this latter form almost invariably elicits a negative response. Related and extremely important areas include history of the menstrual cycle and pregnancies in the female and history of possible urinary or fecal disorders in both sexes. In both sexes, direct and frank questions must be asked in regard to the occurrence of venereal diseases and the use and nature of contraceptive techniques. Insight must be obtained concerning the relationship with "significant others" (Bardach, 1978), whether spouses, companions, or friends. It is essential to obtain a precise idea of the patient's premorbid image of himself or herself in terms of male or female identity.

The elements of physical examination most relevant to sexual problems include inspection, rectal and (in the female) pelvic examination, sensory testing of the saddle (S_2 to S_5) area including the genital areas, and observation of the lumbosacral reflexes. During rectal examination, the observer should note the tone of the anal sphincter and the strength of its voluntary contraction. A reflex contraction of the sphincter is usually obtained on insertion of the palpating finger and by gently applying a pin-prick to the mucocutaneous junction (rectal reflex). In the male, gentle stroking of the glans penis will produce, in the majority of cases, a brisk contraction of the anal sphincter. This is known as the bulbocavernosus reflex and tests the afferent and efferent branches of the pudendal nerves and their connection in the S_3 to S_4 segments of the spinal cord. The bulbocavernosus reflex can be induced and recorded objectively, and it has been suggested that this provides a more stable and reliable method of evaluating subjects who complain of impotence (Ertekin and Reel, 1976).

Application of a cold object to the scrotum or surrounding areas produces a slow vermicular contraction of the dartos, or tunica dartos, a layer of smooth muscle fibers situated in the superficial fascia of the scrotum. This is known as the scrotal reflex, an ANS reflex which is not accompanied by elevation of the testicle. The scrotal reflex should not be confused with the cremasteric reflex, a superficial cutaneous reflex elicited by stroking the skin of the inner thigh and mediated by the ilioinguinal and genitofemoral nerves through the first and second lumbar segments. The normal response of the cremasteric reflex consists of a contraction of the cremasteric muscle with slow elevation of the testicle.

In patients with a spinal cord lesion, a nociceptive or tactile stimulus anywhere below the level of the lesion will produce flexion of the hip, knee, and ankle. On occasion, this flexion spinal defense reflex may be elicited by extreme passive plantar flexion of the toes or foot (Pierre Marie-Foix sign). At times, contraction may be accompanied by muscular contraction of the abdominal wall, evacuation of the bladder or of the bowels, sweating, reflex erythema, or pilomotor responses; in the male, erection and even ejaculation may be part of this reaction, which Riddoch called mass reflex (Riddoch, 1917; De Jong, 1979).

Since the genital organs and the urinary tract share a sizable part of their innervation, tests of bladder function have a definite role in the evaluation of patients with sexual disorders. One must keep in mind that much information can be gained about bladder function without instrumental tests. A good history, measurement of the amount of urine emitted from a full bladder, and, if indicated, postvoiding catheterization often allow a distinction to be made between various types of bladder disorders. Table 2 summarizes the symptoms and findings in five types of neurogenic bladder (Lapides, 1976). In the *uninhibited bladder*, found in bilateral or more rarely unilateral hemispheric or brainstem lesions, the capacity of the bladder may be moderately reduced (to about 250 cc), and there is no residual urine. There is urgency which may or may not be preceded by hesitancy or frequency. Sensation in this disorder is normal. In the *reflex bladder*, typically found in spinal cord lesions above the sacral segments, the capacity of the bladder is markedly reduced (to 100 cc); again there is no or only very little residual urine. Urgency and frequency are felt, but true sensation from the bladder is absent; in this and other cases with absence of true bladder sensation, patients often have knowledge that their bladder is full by nonspecific sensations, due, for example, to pressure on the diaphragm or abdominal wall. The *autonomic* bladder is caused by lesions of the sacral spinal cord, the conus medullaris, cauda equina, or the pelvic nerves. The patient has neither voluntary nor reflex control of the bladder, and limited voiding occurs as a result of the intrinsic bladder innervation. Capacity is moderately increased (to about 800 cc), and there tends to be a large residual; there is no desire to void except for the feeling of abdominal discomfort. There may be frequency, and there is marked hesitancy; voiding is usually produced by increasing the intraabdominal pressure. No sensation is present in the *sensory bladder*, found in lesions of the sensory pathways (posterior roots of the sacral nerves or posterior column of the spinal cord as typically found in tabes dorsalis), there is marked increase in bladder capacity and a large amount of residual urine. Again, there is no desire to void, but there are frequent emissions of small amounts of urine (overflow incontinence). There is of course, no sensation. Finally, in the *motor bladder*, typically found in poliomyelitis, symptoms and signs are similar to those of the sensory bladder, except that there is normal sensation.

Special tests such as cystourethroscopy, cystometry, and sphincter electromyography (EMG) can provide accurate quantitative data regarding these disorders, but because of the special skill required for these tests and their interpretation, they should be performed only by persons who are experts in the field of neurourology. Once again it

TABLE 2. Summary of symptoms and findings in 5 types of neurogenic bladders[a]

Type	Lesion site	Capacity	Residual	Urgency	Frequency	Hesitancy	Sensation
Uninhibited bladder	UMN Cerebral hemispheres	N or –	0	+	0	0 or +	N
Reflex bladder	UMN Spinal cord (upper segments)	–	0 or +	+	+	0 or +	N or –
Autonomic bladder	LMN Spinal cord (lower segments)	+	++	0	++	+	0
Sensory bladder	LMN Sensory pathways	++	+++	0	++	++	0
Motor bladder	LMN Motor pathways	++	+++	0	++	++	N

[a] UMN = upper motor neuron lesion; LMN = lower motor neuron lesion; 0 = absent; N = unchanged; + = increased; – = decreased.

must be stressed that these tests of bladder and related functions are important because of the close relationship between the innervation of the urinary tract and that of the genital organs. Dysfunction in one of the two systems, however, is not necessarily accompanied by dysfunction in the other.

An objective test, more closely related to sexual function in the male, has been used by Karacan (1970), Fisher and co-workers (1975), and Jovanovic (1967). The method is based on the fact that during sleep, males tend to have penile tumescence as part of the "autonomic storm" that accompanies rapid eye movement (REM) sleep (Fisher et al., 1965; Karacan et al., 1966). Changes in penile circumference can be fairly easily recorded and may provide an objective index of a male's ability to obtain an erection. An objective way of analyzing female erotic response based on vaginal plethysmography has also been described (Sinthack and Geer, 1975).

Since a considerable portion of the innervation of the sexual organs is supplied by the ANS, it may be important to evaluate other components of the autonomic (sympathetic) nervous system with special tests. In the sweating test, perspiration may be provoked by external heat (thermoregulatory sweating) which is centrally mediated, or by the subcutaneous injection of cholinergic drugs such as pilocarpine hydrochloride, which act directly on the sympathetic (cholinergic) postganglionic fibers (drug sweating). Various methods have been described to improve the determination of the areas where sweating occurs. One consists of painting the skin with iodine and dusting the painted areas with starch powder which turns bluish black in the presence of iodine and moisture. Other methods are summarized in De Jong's textbook (1979).

The ANS can also be examined by studying circulatory reflexes, which can be elicited by testing for orthostatic hypotension; changes in posture (from horizontal to vertical) should produce no change in blood pressure, but about one-third of normal persons have a fall of 10 to 15 mm Hg in systolic pressure, whereas the diastolic pressure may rise or fall 5 mm Hg. In patients with orthostatic hypotension there is fall of both systolic and diastolic pressure which may or may not be accompanied by light-headedness or impairment of consciousness.

In the Valsalva maneuver, the patient takes a deep breath and then attempts expiration forcibly, with nose and mouth closed. Figure 8 (top) shows the normal response: phase I shows an increase in blood pressure. In phase II, there is a fall followed by a plateau or a slight rise and an increase in heart rate. Phase III follows the release of intrathoracic pressure and is characterized by an abrupt fall of mean blood pressure. Finally, in phase IV, the systolic blood pressure rises above the resting level within 10 seconds of release in intrathoracic pressure and is complete when the blood pressure returns to the resting level, normally within 90 sec. During the overshoot period bradycardia is usually present.

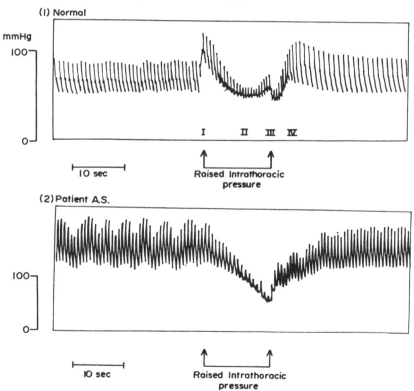

FIG. 8. Blood pressure in a normal subject **(top)** and a patient with orthostatic hypotension **(bottom)** before, during, and after the Valsalva maneuver. The patient's response is blocked. (Reproduced by permission from Johnson RH, and Spalding JMK: *Disorders of the Autonomic Nervous System.* Philadelphia: Davis, 1974.)

Figure 8 (bottom) shows the response of a patient with sympathetic paralysis. Phase II shows a continuing fall of systolic, diastolic, and pulse pressure; heart rate usually increases. On release of intrathoracic pressure (phases III and IV) there is no overshoot and no bradycardia. The blood pressure gradually returns to the resting level.

Another easy way to measure vascular reflexes is by measuring blood pressure response to a sustained handgrip at 30% of maximum voluntary contraction. A rise of more than 16 mm Hg of the diastolic blood pressure is normally seen. A rise of less than 10 mm Hg is considered abnormal (Ewing et al., 1973).

These various test results of autonomic function can be expected to be particularly impaired in patients with diseases that tend to affect the ANS, such as diabetes, amyloidosis, etc. The sweat test may also be used to diagnose the level and completeness of spinal cord lesions. In general it can be stated that an abnormal result in any of the tests mentioned in this section favors an organic cause for symptoms of sexual dysfunction, and should, therefore, stimulate the physician to take further diagnostic steps aimed at eliciting the precise etiology of these symptoms.

Chapter 4

Clinical Syndromes

Many neurological syndromes may produce an impairment of sexual functions, and their classification is undoubtedly difficult. We have chosen to divide these syndromes according to the site of the nervous system where the brunt of the lesion is usually located. It must be kept in mind, however, that many neurological syndromes affect several different systems. For example, diabetes may affect not only the peripheral nerves but practically all other parts of the nervous system as well. Idiopathic orthostatic hypotension is perhaps the most difficult condition to classify anatomically. At times, it affects the spinal cord but many other structures tend to be affected as well. Our anatomical classification, however, arbitrary as it is, appears the most convenient. We shall then separate diseases that affect predominantly the peripheral nerves (peripheral neuropathies) from those that tend to affect predominantly, on one hand, the spinal cord and on the other hand the cerebral hemispheres. A separate section will deal with drugs (since they tend to affect separate parts of the nervous system sometimes simultaneously) and a final one will deal with aging.

PERIPHERAL NEUROPATHIES

Diabetes Mellitus

Diabetes mellitus is a hereditary disease that tends to affect many parts and organs of the body. It is perhaps best known for its effects on carbohydrate, lipid, and protein metabolism secondary to deficient insulin production. Diabetes, however, also tends to produce a vascular syndrome consisting of accelerated atherosclerosis (premature aging) and a specific disease of small vessels (microangiopathy) that affects particularly the kidneys, the eyes, and many other parts of the body including the central and peripheral nervous system. Keeping these facts in mind is essential for an understanding of the effects and for the management of diabetes mellitus.

It has been known for many years that sexual difficulties are frequently found in male diabetics and may in fact occasionally be the presenting symptom of the disease. Difficulty with erection is the most common form. According to Rubin and Babbott (1958), this symptom is found in 25% of patients aged 30 to 34, rising to over 50% in the 50- to 54-year-old age group. These figures are two to five times greater than those found in normal controls. The course of impotence with diabetes is usually one of decreased firmness of erection and a gradual onset of impotence over a course of six months. There may also be retrograde ejaculation in the context of normal erection and orgasm (Greene et al., 1963). Priapism also has been occasionally reported (Thomas and Lascelles, 1966). Sexual drive remains intact in practically all patients (Ellenberg, 1971).

Diabetic males who experience difficulty with erection often have a peripheral neuropathy characterized by diminished sensation or by painful sensations, occurring either spontaneously or elicited by touch; there can also be wasting of the muscles and weakness and trophic changes of the skin, joints, and bones. These changes are found mainly in the feet and legs. Their cause is unclear; there is no correlation between the severity of the disease and the progression of polyneuropathy, and symptoms of neuropathy may occur in diabetic patients whose blood sugar levels have been well controlled.

Ellenberg (1971) found a peripheral neuropathy in 38 of 45 patients with impotence. Martin (1953), on the other hand, found that only one-half of his patients with neuropathy were impotent. This suggests that impotence in diabetic males is not directly related to peripheral neuropathy.

Because of the strong dependence of sexual function on normal parasympathetic and sympathetic activity (see pp. 11–17), impairment of the ANS would be expected to be a frequent correlate of impotence in diabetic males. It is certainly true that a proportion of these patients also complain of orthostatic hypotension, diarrhea, and difficulty with micturition. Ellenberg (1971) performed cystometrograms in 45 diabetic males who complained of impotence and obtained normal findings in only 8 cases. His other 37 patients had abnormal cystometrograms with increased bladder capacity (i.e., greater than 500 cc). Six patients also had residual urine and yet no bladderneck obstruction was shown cystoscopically. Two patients with impotence and an abnormal cystometrogram showed a normal peripheral nervous system on clinical examination. Five of the diabetic patients had neither cystometric abnormalities nor involvement of the peripheral nervous system; Ellenberg concluded that impotence was psychogenic in at least four of the five "as indicated by the presence of morning erections and competence in extramarital situation in two and intermittent impotence in two." In contrast, 3 of 30 diabetics without complaints of impotence had abnormal cystometrograms.

Ewing and co-workers (1973) studied the vascular reflexes of the ANS of 37 diabetic patients (6 females, 31 males) having symptoms suggestive of autonomic neuropathy. Of the 31 males, 28 complained of impotence, an isolated symptom in 15 of the men. They did not comment on the symptoms of their female patients. Fourteen patients had postural hypotension. Vascular reflexes were studied by recording heart-rate changes during the Valsalva maneuver and by measuring blood pressure response to sustained handgrip in 15 patients. There was a low ($r = 0.36$) correlation between the results of the two tests. All patients with postural hypotension had an abnormal Valsalva response. Patients with abnormal vascular reflexes had greater evidence of peripheral neuropathies as measured by nerve conduction studies. There was a striking difference in responses between the patients with impotence alone and those with other features of autonomic neuropathy with or without impotence. The 15 patients whose impotence was the only manifestation suggestive of diabetic autonomic neuropathy had less abnormal vascular reflexes than did the rest of the patients, who had other features of diabetic autonomic neuropathy. Ewing and his co-workers (1973) concluded that only when impotence is associated with other features of the disorder can it be reliably attributed to autonomic neuropathy. These findings suggest that when other evidence of autonomic neuropathy is absent, the clinician would do well to explore other possible causes of sexual dysfunction including concurrent medical diseases of other types, medications being taken by the patient, and finally, psychological or interpersonal problems being experienced by the patient.

A more direct method of measurement was applied by Karacan and co-workers (1978) to a) 35 diabetic men who complained of impotence and who were seeking implantation of a penile prosthesis and b) 35 age-matched normal controls. Seven diabetics were found to have normal noctural penile tumescence (NPT) (i.e., at least one episode of normal NPT per night), and the other twenty-eight had either abnormally diminished or absent NPT.

Low and co-workers (1975) performed a pathology study of the greater splanchnic nerve of 8 known diabetic patients (ages 31 to 71). In 5, sural nerves were also studied. Comparison with age-matched nondiabetic controls showed that in diabetics the fiber density of the greater splanchnic nerve was greatly reduced; fiber density was also reduced in the sural nerves. It is not known whether these patients were impotent or had other symptoms or signs of ANS dysfunction. The functional implications of these findings are, therefore, unclear but they suggest a structural alteration of autonomic nerves as the pathological basis of various autonomic disorders of diabetics including orthostatic hypotension and impotence.

Despite this indirect evidence that impotence may be due to a neuropathy affecting the ANS, other potential causes have been investigated. The possible etiological role of hormonal disorders has been discussed (Schoffling et al., 1963), but most authors tend to attribute little importance to it, particularly in view of normal testosterone levels in these patients (Kolodny, Kahn, Goldstein, et al., 1974). However, some evidence suggests that erectile competence may depend on a more complex set of hormonal values and, even in the absence of other physical or psychological problems, may well be influenced by more than simply the testosterone level. There still remains a certain number of diabetics in whom the etiology of the impotence is unclear.

The sexual behavior of diabetic females has received much less attention than that of males. Kolodny (1971) reviewed the sexual history of 125 female diabetics compared with that of 100 hospitalized nondiabetic females in the same age group. Only women with admitted coital activity during the previous year were included in this study. Of the 125 diabetic women, 44 (35.2%) reported complete absence of orgasmic response during the year preceding inquiry; only 6 of the 100 nondiabetic women had failed to achieve orgasm. None of the nonorgasmic women without diabetes had ever previously experienced orgasm, whereas 40 of the 44 nonorgasmic diabetic women had been orgasmic in the past and had developed a pattern of sexual dysfunction following the onset of diabetes.

There was little correlation between age at the time of the study and sexual dysfunction. There was no significantly greater evidence of more severe diabetes (as measured by insulin dose, retinopathy, neuropathy, nephropathy, or vaginitis) in those diabetics with impaired sexual function than in the sexually normal diabetic women. The only result that could suggest a causative factor was the striking correlation between duration of diabetes and frequency of sexual dysfunction.

Later studies have shown that evidence of ANS involvement can be found in some diabetic women (Brooks, 1977). In a recent review, Kolodny and co-workers (1979) have suggested that in addition to possible neurological damage, other elements may play an important role in the sexual dysfunctions of diabetic women. These include greater susceptibility to infection, particularly vaginal infections and, in some cases, fear of the complications of pregnancy associated with diabetes or concern about the increased risk of congenital defects in children. These may well predispose the female diabetic to the development of psychogenic sexual difficulties.

Treatment

The therapy for sexual inadequacy in male diabetics varies according to the specific etiology. Occasionally, impotence in acute diabetes is due to malnutrition and weakness; in such cases, proper general medical management will restore sexual functions. The possible effect of drugs and endocrine factors should always be kept in mind. A possible psychogenic cause of the disorder should be given serious consideration in all cases (Ellenberg, 1978). Frequently, men who have inherited the disorder from fathers or grandfathers, known by them to have become impotent in later life, assume that their fate will be the same. Likewise, a diabetic male who has not been told that this is likely to be a concomitant of the disorder may suddenly develop impotence when he discovers that diabetics frequently suffer from erectile failure. In both of these cases the problem can be conceptualized as one of performance anxiety and be treated effectively from this conceptual framework.

Prognosis tends to be quite poor when the cause is neurogenic. It is well known that there is little correlation between severity of other diabetic manifestations and sexual difficulties, and in most instances treatment of diabetes fails to restore sexual functions.

Penile prostheses have been advocated in several conditions but have received the greatest attention by workers involved with impotent diabetic males, probably because these patients tend to have normal sex drives and in general do not have motor deficits that might otherwise interfere with coitus. The various types of penile prostheses, and their indications and limitations have been thoughtfully reviewed by Renshaw (1978). For the married patient requesting penile prosthesis, some consideration should be given to the impact of restored sexual function on the marital relationship. A diagnostic interview or consultation interview of the female partner and of both partners as a couple should be considered a requirement prior to surgery. Management of female diabetics with special dysfunctions follows some of the principles that apply to males and consists essentially of careful evaluation and counseling (Kolodny et al., 1979).

Amyloidosis

Amyloid is a fibrous protein that may accumulate extracellularly in various tissues of the body. Amyloidosis may be defined as a condition in which amyloid accumulates in amounts that interfere with normal body functions. Cohen (1980) proposes the following classification of amyloidosis: 1) primary amyloidosis (not associated with pre- or co-existing disease), 2) amyloidosis associated with multiple myeloma, 3) secondary amyloidosis associated with chronic infections (e.g., tuberculosis) or inflammatory diseases (e.g., rheumatoid arthritis), 4) heredofamilial amyloidosis, 5) local amyloidosis, and 6) amyloidosis associated with aging.

Involvement of the ANS and subsequent impotence are particularly prominent in heredofamilial amyloidosis. Impotence can, in fact, be the presenting symptom in such cases, and amyloidosis must therefore be kept in mind in the differential diagnosis of sexual dysfunctions. Of the hereditary amyloidoses, impotence appears to be particularly prominent in those forms with neuropathies affecting predominantly the lower limbs, namely the Portuguese, Japanese, and Swedish type (Cohen and Benson, 1975). In all forms, a pathology examination will show deposits of amyloid in the ANS (Nordborg et al., 1973). It is not known whether sexual dysfunctions are found in females with amyloidosis. The course of generalized amyloidosis is usually slowly progressive. The major cause of death is renal failure. There is no specific therapy for any form of amyloidosis (Cohen, 1980).

Familial Dysautonomia (Reiley-Day Syndrome)

This condition affects the ANS and other parts of the nervous system. The majority of patients are Jewish, of Ashkenazi extraction originating from Eastern Europe. It is arbitrarily discussed here, despite the fact that pathology can be found in several components of the nervous system. The disturbance of the ANS leads to vasomotor changes affecting the skin, fluctuations in blood pressure (hyper- or hypotension), erratic temperature control, hyperhydrosis, diminished or absent lacrimation, and diarrhea and constipation (Johnson and Spalding, 1974). There may also be insensitivity to pain and loss of reflexes. This disease usually affects children, but the few men who survive until maturity tend to be impotent (Young et al., 1975).

Uremic Neuropathy

Patients with chronic renal diseases are frequently impotent, particularly those undergoing dialysis (Sherman, 1975). Uremic neuropathy and, more importantly, hormonal factors, play a significant role in the etiology of the decreased sexual desire and activity observed in both males and females with uremia (Holdsworth, 1977; Bailey, 1977). In a recent study of patients on home dialysis, Stauffer and co-workers (1980) found that while none of the male patients had had erectile problems prior to uremia, 36% reported difficulty getting an erection after the onset of uremia. Among the female patients, difficulty with both arousal and orgasm developed in 11% of them following uremia, and nearly 25% reported insufficient vaginal lubrication.

Other Neuropathies

There are many causes and types of polyneuropathies (Dyck et al., 1975), but in most of them impotence either does not occur very often or occurs only when the patient is so ill that it is very low on the patient's list of problems. This certainly seems to apply to the Guillain-Barré syndrome, porphyria, multiple myeloma, as well as toxicity from exogenous agents such as arsenic or other metals. A noticeable exception, alcohol, will be dealt with in the section on drugs (p. 70). With very few doubtful exceptions (Thomas and Schields, 1970), paraneoplastic neuropathies do not cause prominent disorders of sexual function. Two patients with hemophilia and peripheral neuropathy recently were reported to be impotent (Berry, 1975).

SPINAL CORD LESIONS

Spinal Cord Injuries in Males

Sexual dysfunction following spinal cord injuries has attracted considerable attention from workers in the field and is covered in some detail in the current literature, probably in large part because many of the people affected by spinal cord injury are young, active, and otherwise healthy. Modern techniques of rehabilitation and prosthesis have given them a much greater life expectancy and considerably greater mobility. The Veterans Administration, with its several large Spinal Cord Injury Services, and the British National Spinal Injury Centers have undoubtedly contributed a great deal to our knowledge in this area of sexual dysfunction.

Experts agree that preoccupation with future sexual performance occurs early and is quite prominent in the mind of persons with spinal cord injury. It is, however, imperative for a physician to wait before expressing a prognosis in these cases. When a patient comes to the emergency room with a spinal cord injury, more urgent problems must be dealt with initially, such as assuring urinary flow and avoiding infection. Above all, injuries to the spinal cord tend to be followed acutely by spinal shock which includes complete or almost complete suppression of reflex activity at all spinal cord levels below the lesion (Adams and Victor, 1981). In the male, genital reflexes (reflex penile erection, bulbocavernosus and scrotal reflexes) and in both sexes contraction of the rectal sphincter are abolished or profoundly depressed after such injury. The duration of the spinal shock varies, with some reflexes returning within 1 to 6 weeks. Simply informing patients of the existence of this phenomenon and explaining that an accurate prognosis cannot be arrived at for some time may provide considerable reassurance.

When spinal shock has subsided, two main factors affect the prognosis of future sexual functions: 1) the level of the spinal cord lesion and 2) whether the lesion is a complete or an incomplete one. Incidentally, it must be noted that even in cases of complete lesions, the spinal cord is rarely cut in two, and the piaarachnoid usually is not lacerated. Pathology usually shows traumatic necrosis of the spinal cord (Adams and Victor, 1981). Therefore, use of the term complete lesion or complete section usually refers to a functional concept rather than to a strictly anatomical one.

As pointed out by Tarabulcy (1972), spinal cord injuries affect sexual functions more than they do micturition, which in turn is more vulnerable than defecation. In various series gathered from the literature and comprising 1296 male patients with spinal cord lesions in all segments, Tarabulcy found that erection was preserved in 77%, coitus was possible in 35%, and ejaculation occurred in 10%; 3.4% of patients claimed progeny.

Lesions of the Cauda Equina or Conus Medullaris (Sacral Spinal Cord)

The cauda equina, the name given to the nerve roots at the level of the second lumbar spinal vertebra and below, is obviously not part of the spinal cord, and clinical differentiation between lesions of the cauda and the conus is sometimes possible (De Jong, 1979), usually with less severe and sudden impairment in lesions of the cauda than that of the conus. Nevertheless, the marked similarities between the syndromes are sufficient to warrant their discussion together. They may be caused by penetrating wounds but are more often due to tumors and other space-occupying lesions. The effects on sexual behavior of lesions at this level are the most severe and the least reversible (Piera, 1973). As a rule, patients with lesions in either the conus (sacral spinal cord) or the cauda equina have complete loss of erection, although ejaculation may occasionally occur; they also present with an autonomic bladder (see p. 28), loss of tone in their anal sphincter, absent anal reflex, and loss of tone of the external urethral sphincter.

Lumbar Spinal Cord Lesions

In this group, even complete lesions do not necessarily preclude some type of sexual activity. In one recent series (Comarr, 1975) 20 patients had complete, lower-motor-neuron-type lesions of the cord. Sexual performance was studied in terms of occurrence of erections (divided into psychogenic, spontaneous, and reflex from penile stimulation), coitus (attempted and successful or unsuccessful), ejaculation, and orgasm. Eight patients were able to attain psychogenic erection but none had reflex-stimulated erection. Seven successfully attempted coitus, and five of these achieved ejaculation with orgasm. These positive sexual phenomena were probably mediated via the sympathetic nervous system, the preganglionic fibers of which leave the spinal cord at the lower thoracic and upper lumbar level.

Thoracic and Cervical Spinal Cord Lesions

Lesions in the spinal cord above the lumbar level, when complete, drastically interfere with psychogenic erections; in contrast, however, spontaneous erections are quite common, as is reflex-stimulated erection. Coitus is therefore possible in a certain percentage of cases. Erection, however, is usually short-lived, there is usually no seminal emission, and orgasm is rarely achieved. The fertility of male paraplegics is decreased even in cases in which seminal emission or ejaculation occurs because sperm counts in these patients show only few mobile sperm. The cause of the decrease in sperm production is not known but is believed to be due to intercurrent infections or to impairment of temperature regulation in the scrotum (Appenzeller, 1976).

Spinal Cord Injuries in Females

Sexual problems in female paraplegics have been investigated to a lesser extent than in males (Griffith and Trieschmann, 1975). The problems in females appear to be different from those of males; sensation during intercourse is often absent, and there is a greater frequency of urinary tract infections. In females, the effect of spinal cord injuries on the motor reflexes involved in coitus is unclear; it has been said that vaginal secretions remain active as part of the genital reflex (Griffith and Trieschmann, 1975). One study has suggested that sexual activity continues or may even increase following disability (Weiss and Diamond, 1966). Guttman (1969) stated that, although "typical" orgasm during intercourse is absent in women with complete spinal cord lesions, heightened arousal may be obtained by means of intense tactile stimulation involving parts of the body innervated by spinal cord segments situated above the lesion and, therefore, intact. This seems to be particularly true for the region around the breast for women with a lesion below T_4. Kolodny and co-workers (1979) mention the case of a female who was studied in the Masters and Johnson Institute before and after an injury which affected her spinal cord at the T_{12} level that occurred several years after initial testing. Physiologic studies suggested that in this woman, there had been "transfer of erotic zones from one region of the body (the vagina) to another (the breasts)."

Menstruation tends to be irregular soon after the injury but later returns to normal (Talbot, 1955). In contrast to what happens in male paraplegics, spinal cord injuries above the sacral segments, whether complete or incomplete, do not interfere with women's fertility. There are many cases of women paraplegics who have become pregnant and delivered one or more children normally. In one review of 187 preg-

nancies in female paraplegics (Goller and Paeslack, 1972), the number
of spontaneous first trimester abortions was found to be no greater than
normal, but there was a slight increase in the number of premature
babies weighing less than 2,500 g (only 12% of pregnancies lasted more
than 6 months). There are considerably more complications in women
who become paraplegic during pregnancy. Rossier and co-workers
(1969) pointed out some of the special problems of delivery in paraplegic
women, particularly the need to distinguish autonomic hypereplexia
from preeclampsia or toxemia of pregnancy. Autonomic hypereplexia
is a self-limiting condition, whereas toxemia of pregnancy may be fatal
if not properly treated. Treatment of the most severe cases of eclampsia
is immediate termination of the pregnancy.

Treatment

The practical management of sexual disorders in patients with spinal
cord injuries has been reviewed by several authors (e.g., Trieschmann,
1978). Treatment emphasizes various types of sexual counseling
aimed at affecting attitudes toward sexuality of both patients and their
sexual partners (Eisenberg and Rastad 1976). As pointed out by Trieschmann (1978), and Higgins (1979), although participants in these counseling programs evaluate them positively, no data are available as to
the effectiveness of these programs in changing sexual behavior in
persons with spinal injury. It should be mentioned, however, that to
equate the value of such programs with measurable changes in sexual
behavior, may not be valid. It is possible that the changes that occur
in self-awareness and/or self-acceptance are much more important to
the patient with a spinal cord injury than an increase in the frequency
of sexual intercourse. Finally, Golji (1979) has reported on the results
of penile prosthesis implantation in 20 spinal-cord-injured males who
were followed between 3 and 27 months postoperatively. All patients
reported increased sexual satisfaction for themselves and their partners
and 18 of 20 patients wished they had had the implant earlier.

Poliomyelitis

This disease, even though it has almost disappeared in North America
and Western Europe, has remained endemic in other parts of the world.

Poliomyelitis is a viral disease that affects mainly the anterior horns of the spinal cord and therefore produces an impairment of the voluntary movements. It usually produces little direct interference with the functioning of sexual organs; impotence, when it occurs, is generally transient. A more serious problem is posed by poliomyelitis that complicates pregnancy. Pratt and co-workers (1958) suggested that in such cases a caesarean section will not only save a viable fetus but may also, coincidentally, improve the mother's condition. This, however, may not be always true. Benson *(personal communication)* reports the case of a female who developed severe poliomyelitis during her pregnancy. She had to be kept in a respirator constantly, and great care was taken by the medical staff to be ready to support both the patient and the infant at the time of delivery. All their preparations were useless, however, as the patient delivered precipitously in the elevator on the way to the delivery room. Subsequently, both mother and child did excellently.

Syphilis

Like poliomyelitis, syphilis of the nervous system has become a rare condition in North America and Western Europe, but remains a frequent problem in some other parts of the world (Evans, 1976). Neurosyphilis, one of the manifestations of tertiary syphilis, can be subdivided into tabes dorsalis (affecting mainly the spinal roots and cord) and general paresis. In tabes dorsalis, impotence may occur as part of a loss of spinal reflexes due to interruption of the afferent arc or reflex, a phenomenon that also brings about an autonomic bladder and orthostatic hypotension (Sharpey-Shafer, 1956). Erection disorders occur in 27% of males; because of lack of sensitivity or other disorders, sexual performance is also impaired in 8% of females (Alpers and Mancall, 1971). Another complication of tabes dorsalis that seriously interferes with sexuality is the occurrence of priapism (Becker and Mitchell, 1965). Sexual functions in patients with general paresis have not been studied.

Vascular Lesions

Vascular lesions may occasionally produce spinal cord lesions which resemble, from the point of view of subsequent sexual dysfunction, those of complete or incomplete spinal cord injury. In the Leriche syndrome (Leriche and Morel, 1948) (atherosclerotic occlusion of the iliac arteries), the spinal cord is not affected, but impotence is a prominent sequela due to decreased blood supply to the genital organs and perhaps also because of a lesion to peripheral structures, such as the superior hypogastric sympathetic plexus. The latter structure may also be affected in the course of aortoiliac reconstructive surgery (Sabri and Cotton, 1971).

Idiopathic Orthostatic Hypotension

Idiopathic orthostatic hypotension was originally described by Bradbury and Eggelston (1925; 1927), but is often referred to as Shy-Drager syndrome (Shy and Drager, 1960). As indicated previously, this condition affects various parts of the nervous system and its inclusion in the category of spinal cord disorders is quite arbitrary. It mainly affects middle-aged men with symptoms consisting of loss of sweating, sphincter disturbance, and orthostatic hypotension. Impotence (mainly failure of erection) occurs early and fairly uniformly. Autopsy usually reveals marked cell loss in the intermediolateral column of the thoracolumbar spinal cord. In many cases, autonomic failure is accompanied by multiple system degeneration. Both clinically and pathologically, these patients tend to show either olivo-ponto-cerebellar degeneration or parkinsonism. This topic is well reviewed in the literature (Barns et al., 1971; Johnson and Spalding, 1974; Appenzeller, 1976).

Multiple Sclerosis

Multiple Sclerosis (MS) is a fairly common CNS disease that affects mainly young adults. Although epidemiological studies have suggested that a virus may be involved in MS, its etiology remains unknown, and only symptomatic treatment is available at the present time. The disease is characterized by loss of myelin in the white matter of the brain, brainstem, and spinal cord and is therefore part of a group of conditions known as demyelinating diseases. The percentage of males with MS and impaired sexual functions is quite high. Impotence occurred in 26%

of patients and was the presenting symptom in 7% of 54 males with MS studied at the Mayo clinic (Ivers and Goldstein, 1963). In one of the most detailed studies on this subject, Vas (1969) studied 37 male patients 18 to 50 years of age. Criteria for inclusion in the study included clearly established MS, ability to walk and be up and about for at least 12 hours, and normal libido. Sixteen patients (43%) were either totally or partially impotent, i.e., gave a history of absent or deficient penile erection. This symptom was more frequent and more severe in patients who had the disease for the longest time; for example, patients with total impotence had had MS for an average of 12 years, while the men with normal potency had had the disease for an average of 5.5 years. Impotent men had a greater incidence of sensory and bowel-bladder abnormalities. Studies of the autonomic functions of these men showed no orthostatic hypotension in any subject. There was, however, a relationship between impotence and anhydrosis (loss of sweating); the totally impotent patients did not perspire below the iliac crests; the partially impotent patient would sweat on the face, upper limbs, trunk, and perineum, but not on the lower limbs. The integrity of the postganglionic sympathetic fibers and the presence of sweat glands in the dry skin areas were confirmed by administration of intradermal acetylcholine and intravenous pilocarpine. Lumbosacral reflexes (scrotal, bulbocavernosus, and rectal reflexes) were absent in all 3 totally impotent patients, absent in some of the partially impotent men, but intact in almost all the normally potent men. The authors concluded that impotence in patients with MS is due to lesions of the spinal cord in its thoracolumbar segments. Interestingly, Vas (1969) observed that during the length of this study, sexual potency tended to remit and relapse in 4 patients with a corresponding change in the pattern of sweating. This finding of oscillating sexual function in MS patients could have important implications for the counseling of such patients with respect to their sexuality. Since the patient who becomes impotent may interpret this as a totally permanent change unless otherwise instructed, simply having the information that sexual function may return even temporarily can have a positive impact on the patient's self-image if not on functioning itself.

Comparable results have been obtained by Cartlidge (1972), who also found that 7 of 20 patients with MS were impotent and had impaired sweating but normal Valsalva maneuver and no orthostatic hypotension. He concluded that vasomotor and sudomotor pathways may be separated, and that sudomotor function is a more sensitive index of autonomic function than are blood vessel responses.

Sexual functions of females with MS have been studied recently by Lilius and co-workers (1976) and by Lundberg (1978). Lilius and colleagues found, on the basis of a written questionnaire, that 39% of females and 64% of males reported sexual difficulties. Many of these patients were at a fairly advanced stage of the disease, but Lundberg, who studied women who were at an earlier stage and were experiencing little or no physical disability, found sexual problems in 13 of 25 women (52%). Symptoms included decreased libido, difficulty with orgasmic response, dyspareunia, and, in 3 patients, lack of vaginal lubrication. Many authors think that MS in females is made worse by pregnancy and lactation (see McAlpine et al., 1972, for a discussion).

Group counseling of MS patients has recently been described (Hartings et al., 1976). This approach may be particularly valuable in discussing sexual dysfunction in patients with MS.

Other Spinal Cord Diseases

In the myelopathy of cervical spondylosis, one of the conspicuous features of the typical clinical picture is the absence of impairment of sphincter control and sexual functions (Brain and Wilkinson, 1967). In amyotrophic lateral sclerosis, sexual functions are not affected directly. In fact, the normal desire and normal functioning of the sex organs often contrast with the severely reduced motor power; this disproportion may add an additional disturbing feature to the disease (Special Correspondent, 1971). As indicated above, lateral cordotomies performed for treatment of intractable pain may interfere with erection in the male, especially if the procedure is performed bilaterally (Olivecrona, 1947).

HEMISPHERIC LESIONS

As stated earlier, very little is known of the anatomy and clinical physiology of the pathways that connect the spinal cord and peripheral innervation of the sexual organs with the higher centers. This is probably due to the fact that in the brainstem, for example, the responsible structures and pathways are in very close contact with many others that give more obvious clinical manifestations and tend perhaps to obscure the observation of sexual disorders. We have slightly better knowledge of the relationship between the cerebral hemispheres (particularly the cortex) and sexual functions, probably because the corresponding areas are large and because specific areas tend to be separated. This and the fact that some lesions are limited to discrete areas of the brain have contributed a great deal to our knowledge of the role played in behavior by specific cortical areas.

From the foregoing, one can see that in the field of changes in sexual behavior (as in practically every other behavioral change of neurological origin), the emphasis should be not so much on the pathological type of cerebral lesion but on its localization. The main areas of the human brain known for their relation to sexual behavior are the frontal and temporal lobes. More limited knowledge has been derived from the study of patients with lesions of subcortical areas.

Subcortical Structures

On the basis of electrical stimulation of the brain carried out to treat a variety of psychiatric and neurological disorders, Heath (1964, 1977), postulated that activity of the corticomedial amygdala and the septal region (Heath and Harper, 1976) correlates with pleasurable emotions. Penile erections were noted in 3 patients during electrical stimulation and orgasmic response was reported by 1 female patient during chemical stimulation of the septal area (Heath, 1964). Isolated lesions of these areas are certainly not frequent in humans. A patient of Poeck and Pilleri (1965), a female in her early 20s, may be an illustration of irritative lesions in this general area. She developed periodic release of aggressive and hypersexual behavior characterized by frequent masturbation, self-reports of markedly increased sex urge, and openly seductive behavior. She was found at autopsy to have encephalitis (resembling von Economo's lethargic encephalitis) with rather extensive lesions of limbic midline structures. Nathan (1969, p. 198) briefly mentions a similar case. Lesions in that area may also be responsible for the hypersexual behavior noted in some patients with deep frontotemporal tumors (Anastasopoulos, 1958) and rabies (Gastaut and Mileto, 1954).

Meyers (1963) reported 4 patients (3 males and 1 female) who developed marked and sustained decrease in sexual drive and, in the case of the males, impotence, following bilaterally homologous surgical interruption of the ansa lenticularis. A fifth patient who underwent bilaterally nonhomologous two-staged ansotomy did not develop sexual impairment. Meyers (1961) attributed the observed decrease in sexual behavior to interruption of a central mechanism located in the septofornicohypothalamic region.

Patients with Parkinson's disease tend to have impaired sexual functions as well as urinary symptoms. The latter have been studied to some extent (Porter and Bors, 1971), but the precise prevalence and pathophysiology of decreased sexual functions is unclear. Several potential factors could be responsible, particularly mental depression and impaired movements. Whether there is a more specific effect of the disease, possibly related to its biochemical abnormalities (decrease in dopamine), remains unknown (Barbeau et al., 1971). The alleged improvement of sexual symptoms with dopaminergic drugs will be discussed in the section on drugs (pp. 68–69).

Patients with Huntington's disease do not have specific sexual disorders. Some anecdotal reports of their increased coital frequency and progeny as well as their reported high rate of "abnormal sexual behavior" (Dewhurst et al., 1977) may be related to the disinhibition which bears some resemblance to the "frontal dementia" to be discussed below. In more advanced stages of the disease, there is, of course, interference with sexual behavior by nonspecific symptoms such as abnormal movements and dementia.

The very few data available on sexual behavior of patients with Korsakoff's syndrome suggest that sexual function tends to be absent in the acute phase of the illness, but may return many months after the onset of the illness (Victor et al., 1971).

Frontal Lobes

Two different areas warrant particular discussion, the paracentral lobules and the granular frontal cortex. The paracentral lobules. corresponding to the merging of the precentral (or prerolandic) and post-central (or retrorolandic) gyri on the convexity and over the medial part of each cerebral hemisphere, are like the two gyri of which they form the continuation; the anterior part of the paracentral lobule is related mainly to motion, whereas the posterior part (like the postcentral gyrus) is related mainly to superficial sensation from the lower part of the body. The granular frontal cortex (sometimes called the prefrontal cortex) is the cortex located in the most anterior part of the frontal lobes, in front of the cortex mainly responsible for motion, such as the precentral gyrus. This latter area is sometimes called the agranular frontal cortex because of the prominence of pyramidal cells and its paucity of granules.

Paracentral Lobules

It has been known for some time that electrical stimulation of the posterior portion of the paracentral lobules in humans produces sensation related to the genital area. Stimulation of the anterior part does not produce motion such as penile erection, but it may produce contraction of the rectal sphincter (Penfield and Rasmussen, 1950). Seizures due to epileptic foci located in the paracentral lobules (Bancaud et al., 1970) consist mainly of lateralized genital paraesthesias (abnormal sensations) at the level of the penis or vagina, rectum, anus, abdomen, etc. These abnormal sensations tend to have little sexual resonance. Erickson (1945) described a female patient with a hemangioma of the paracentral lobule who experienced paraesthesias of this kind; reference to these as "erotomania" is probably misleading.

Granular Frontal Cortex

It has long been known that some patients with frontal lobe pathology involving the "prefrontal" areas tend to show disinhibition and may in fact be brought to the attention of physicians or authorities because of abnormally impulsive sexual behavior. Not all patients with frontal lobe lesions show this picture. As noted by Blumer and Benson (1975), two types of personality changes (frontal dementias) may be described following frontal lobe lesions. One tends toward apathy, depression, or indifference (pseudodepressed type), the other toward apathy, puerility, and euphoria (pseudopsychopathic type). They argue that the pseudodepressed type is found in lesions of the convexity of the frontal lobes, while the pseudopsychopathic type follows lesions of the orbital surface. Bilateral lesions are probably necessary to produce marked personality changes. Abnormal disinhibited social (including sexual) behavior is most commonly found in the pseudopsychopathic type. Pathology may be posttraumatic (Harlow, 1868), infectious (e.g., in general paresis), or tumoral (Weinstein, 1974). Patients with Huntington's disease or MS may occasionally show this type of disorder.

Sequelae of Frontal Lobotomies

Before World War II, Moniz (1937) proposed that a surgical procedure consisting of ablating part of the frontal lobes was successful in relieving symptoms of schizophrenia and other psychiatric disorders. This procedure has now been largely abandoned. Most patients who have undergone frontal leucotomy show either normal or, more often, decreased libido. For example, in a long-term follow-up study, Partridge (1960) found that of 300 patients with prefrontal leucotomy, only 3 had experienced increased libido. Based on follow-up of 3,400 patients who had been subjected to frontal lobotomy, Freeman (1973) noticed that surgery (which tends to be performed on patients who, as part of their severe emotional distress were hyposexual) is "often followed, at least temporarily, by increased libido" but that "only occasionally does it result in disconcerting or annoying demands for sexual gratification."

Temporal Lobes

Temporal Lobe Epilepsy

Much of what we know about the relations between the temporal lobe and sexual behavior derives from clinical observations and occasionally neurosurgical intervention in patients with epilepsy (Blumer and Walker, 1975; Rosenblum, 1974). Attention has recently been drawn to the analogy (for the outside observer) between epilepsy and sex expressed by the Latin saying "Coitus brevis epilepsia est." The mood of sexual desire is likened to the prodrome of an epileptic attack, the premonition of orgasm to the aura, and the sexual climax to the epileptic paroxysm. A refractory period, reduced tension, and sleep tend to follow the sex act and the epileptic attack (Blumer and Walker, 1975). It is, however, focal temporal lobe epilepsy that has, to a great extent, contributed to our knowledge of the relevance of specific areas of the human cortex to sexuality. A discussion of sexual behavior in temporal lobe epileptics may be clarified by a distinction between ictal behavior (i.e., occurring during seizures), postictal behavior (i.e., occurring immediately following seizures) and interictal behavior (i.e., behavior between paroxysmal episodes).

Ictal Behavior

An uncommon but well-documented occurrence is that of the sexual seizures found in patients in whom there is paroxysmal abnormal sexual arousal at the time of their seizure. Bancaud and co-workers (1970) found 29 cases in the literature with temporal lobe lesions. The behavior of these patients during seizures has similarities with behavior during masturbation or intercourse, and these may be an orgasm-like sensation. Additional cases have been reported by Currier and co-workers (1971). Himmelhoch and Detre *(unpublished data)* point out that in patients who do show sexual-like behavior during ictus, such seizures are often misdiagnosed as hysterical in origin. This is especially disturbing, since when such seizures have been observed, they were frequently found to result from tumors or other serious medical illness.

As is the case with the majority of patients with temporal lobe epilepsy (King and Ajmone Marsan, 1977), patients with sexual seizures often experience subjective phenomena (aura) during the preictal stage. These include epigastric sensation, abdominal pain, or olfactory sensations. Before and during the seizure there may be fear or paradoxical painful experiences. Conversely, Hoenig and Hamilton (1960) have reported a patient whose epileptic seizures were triggered by sexual orgasm. Gautier-Smith (1980) has recently reported a similar case of a 28-year-old nurse who developed seizures related to her first orgasm. The author attributes these seizures to the hyperventilation that accompanied that sexual experience.

Postictal Sexual Arousal

Blumer (1970) reported cases of postictal sexual arousal in which transient hypersexuality followed an epileptic attack. These episodes differed from the usual postictal phenomena in that they were usually fully remembered by the patients. Blumer also noted that postictal hypersexuality was found "only in those patients who were somehow sexually active." This was also true for ictal hypersexuality and for patients with increased sexual arousal due to seizure control with medication (drug-induced hypersexuality). The implication of this finding is that patients who are interictally hyposexual (as is true for the great majority of patients with temporal lobe epilepsy) are unlikely to show a reversal of that impairment during or after a seizure.

Interictal Sexual Behavior

An early study of the interictal sexual behavior of patients with temporal lobe epilepsy (Gastaut and Collomb, 1954) showed that 24 of 36 patients had sexual difficulties, whereas patients with other types of epilepsy did not. Among the 24 with poor sexual adjustment, the salient quality was decreased sexual drive. Other studies have confirmed that patients with temporal lobe epilepsy definitely tend to be hyposexual. For example, 29 of 42 patients described by Blumer and Walker (1975) had "chronic global hyposexuality," i.e., a markedly decreased frequency of sexual arousal. Temporal lobe epileptics with onset of the illness prior to or at the time of puberty may never or only rarely experience sexual arousal. On the other hand, Hierons and Saunders (1966) and Saunders and Rawson (1970) found that a certain number of patients had normal libido but were impotent. This was present, for example, in 7 patients of Saunders and Rawson (1970) out of a series of 33 with temporal epilepsy, 12 of whom had some sexual disorder; 2 had global hyposexuality, 1 was thought to have psychogenic impotence, 1 was hyposexual but also quite drowsy because of phenobarbital (when phenobarbital was decreased, both his mental status and sexual behavior returned to normal). Only 1 patient of Saunders and Rawson

(1970) showed doubtful hypersexuality, a phenomenon rarely observed by other authors.

Temporal Lobectomies

The effect of temporal lobectomy on sexual behavior was studied by Blumer and Walker (1967) in 21 patients with temporal lobe epilepsy who underwent unilateral temporal lobectomies. Eleven of these patients had become markedly hyposexual following the onset of seizures. Four patients who had a marked decrease in seizures showed lasting improvement in sexual drive. Three patients had a temporary improvement of their seizures, during which time there was an increase in sex drive; return of the seizures coincided with a marked decrease in libido. Finally, in 4 patients hyposexuality persisted; 2 had no improvement in their seizures, 1 had a slight improvement, and 1 had been relieved of his seizures. In another series (Taylor, 1969), 100 patients (63 men and 37 women) were subjected to anterior temporal lobectomy for epilepsy. Following the operation, 22 patients improved their rating of sexual adjustment, but 14 became worse. Fourteen remained in good adjustment, whereas 50 remained poorly adjusted. Here again the most frequent abnormality was low sexual drive, not a failure of erection or ejaculation. Only 1 patient, a female, had an "excessive heterosexual appetite."

Since temporal lobe epilepsy often affects only one side of the brain, it would be of interest to find out if unilateral temporal lobe seizures and unilateral temporal lobectomies have different consequences on sexual behavior according to the affected hemisphere. There is little evidence to support the assumption that they do. Taylor (1969) does not mention laterality but Blumer and Walker (1967) specifically state that laterality of the lesion was of no importance relative to the sexual response of their patients studied before and after unilateral temporal lobectomy. In another line of research, Bear and Fedio (1977) assessed specific personality traits in 27 patients with unilateral temporal lobe epilepsy with a questionnaire completed by both subjects and observers (raters); they found that patients with right-sided lesions tended to deny having sexual alterations. For example, an item exploring unusual sexual practices was denied by all right-temporal-lobe patients, but affirmed by one-third of their raters. This was part of a tendency of these patients to "polish" their own image, whereas left-temporal-lobe patients tended to "tarnish" it by stressing socially unacceptable traits. One could tentatively conclude that the behavioral changes are the same with lesions of either hemisphere, but that frequency of reporting of abnormalities of any kind should be greater with left temporal foci.

The general impression from the material reviewed thus far is that most patients with temporal lobe epilepsy and disorders of sexual behavior tend to be hyposexual, and that temporal lobectomy tends to improve sexual behavior, usually through an increase in libido. Blumer and Walker (1975) implied that this change is mediated by the control of seizures, since "contrary to suspicion, anticonvulsants may reestablish a sexual arousal if they suppress the seizure activity." This is probably not always the case. Saunders and Rawson (1970) noted that patients whose seizures are fairly well controlled by medication may remain hyposexual, and that in some others hyposexuality or impotence may even precede the onset of seizures.

As noted earlier, animal studies have suggested that bilateral temporal lobectomies may produce hypersexuality. This is rarely observed in humans. The most frequently quoted case of Klüver-Bucy syndrome in man (Terzian and Dalle Ore, 1955) was criticized by Appenzeller (1976), who noted that the patient only showed increased erections and tendency to masturbate, a behavior observed in other brain lesions as well, and qualitatively different from what most would consider true hypersexual behavior.

The effect of temporal lobectomy on ictal sexual behavior has been described by Mitchell and co-workers (1954). Their patient used a safety pin as a fetish object. Observing a pin was the only way he could overcome his usual impotence. Whenever the patient used the safety pin to achieve sexual arousal, he had an epileptic seizure. Following a left temporal lobectomy, the sight of a shiny safety pin no longer precipitated seizures, the patient became fully potent, and he no longer had to rely on the fetish for sexual stimulation.

Other Temporal Lobe Lesions

Little information is available about the effect of nonepileptogenic temporal lobe lesions on sexual behavior. This is probably due to the fact that other lesions (e.g., strokes) either do not affect the amygdala and other parts of the limbic system or, if they do, they produce such severe behavioral disruption that sexual functions can no longer be meaningfully observed. It is, however, the authors' personal impression that bilateral temporal lobe lesions tend to depress sexual behavior.

The Effect of Strokes

As previously noted, the sexual sequelae of localized lesions vary markedly according to the nature, size and, above all, location of the lesion. For example, lateral temporal lobe lesions of several different etiologies (traumatic, vascular, infectious, etc.) may closely mimic the interictal sexual changes found in patients with temporal lobe epilepsy as noted in the previous section. Patients with bilateral frontal lesions such as those found in tumors or in general paresis may present with inappropriately disinhibited sexual behavior (Weinstein, 1974). Studies of sexual problems in stroke patients (Renshaw, 1975) show a less specific effect which has been almost completely neglected in the neurological literature. It is true that few physicians follow a sufficiently large number of stroke patients for enough time to gain a clear notion of possible changes in their sexual behavior. Perhaps because of their longer and more personal involvement in patients' rehabilitation, speech pathologists (Malone, 1975) and psychologists (Lezak, 1978) are more likely than doctors to be the confidants of patients and their spouses about personal matters such as their sexual life.

In a recent autobiography relating his recovery from his own stroke, Dahlberg, a psychiatrist, stated "I think that aside from the greater fatigue and the ordinary slowing down that comes with age in man, I am sexually about where I was before the stroke." He went on to add: "I have heard it said that following a stroke, sex is finished. I want to clear up that misapprehension now. It is true, of course, that certain physical difficulties such as hand or leg paralysis might alter sexual athletics, but physical difficulties do not alter orgasmic potential. What may happen, and frequently does, is that emotional depression following a stroke (and most chronic diseases) severely limits sexual as well as any other interest. But this is not a physical disability, and if the emotional depression can be overcome, sexuality can rapidly return to normal and even help alleviate the depression." (Dahlberg and Jaffe, 1977).

Dahlberg noticed, however, that after his stroke there was a decrease in libido and that it was 3 weeks after his stroke that he noticed for the first time he had awakened with an erection. It is important to keep in mind that Dahlberg suffered a relatively mild stroke that had left few sequelae, as shown by the fact that he was able to resume work as a psychiatrist within 20 months of his stroke.

One can wonder about the consequences of strokes on sexual life in the general population. Very few studies have been conducted on this topic. Ford and Orfiren (1976) reported that 60% of stroke patients under the age of 60 stated that their libido had not changed. In a more systematic manner, Kalliomaki and co-workers (1961) also studied patients under the age of 60. Their sample consisted of 105 patients (56 males and 49 females), 36 of whom had suffered from a left-side paralysis, 45 from a right-side paralysis. A cerebrovascular accident without hemiplegia had occurred in 11 and a subarachnoid hemorrhage in 13 cases. Table 3 shows the effect of stroke on libido in the 81 patients in whom the side of the cerebral lesion could be clearly established. As can be seen, a decrease in libido was greater following left-hemisphere lesions (37.8%) than after right-hemisphere lesions (16.7%). This difference was statistically significant ($p < .05$). There was also a greater number of patients with increased libido following lesions of the right hemisphere, but the numbers are quite small and this difference is probably not significant. These researchers also recorded the effect of the stroke on coital frequency. Of 45 males in whom adequate information could be obtained, 34 (76%) had a decrease in coital frequency compared to 11 of 23 females (48%). Only 1 patient (a male with a left-hemisphere lesion) reported increased coital frequency. It is unfortunate that in their brief report Kalliomaki and co-workers (1961) did not specify the criteria used to decide that there had been a change in libido. In a more recent study, Goddess and colleagues (1979) also

TABLE 3. *Effect of cerebral vascular accident on libido[a,b]*

	RH lesions				LH lesions			
	−	+	○	?	−	+	○	?
Males	4	2	15	1	9	1	12	1
Females	2	1	9	2	8	1	8	5
Total	6	3	24	3	17	2	20	6
	16.7	8.3	66.7	8.3	37.8	4.4	44.4	13.4

[a]Table presents data on 36 patients with right hemisphere lesions and 45 patients with left hemisphere lesions.

[b]Legend: RH = right hemisphere; LH = left hemisphere; − = decreased; + = increased; ○ = unchanged; ? = no adequate information.

Modified, from data of Kalliomaki et al (1961).

found that libido was more commonly diminished following strokes affecting the dominant hemisphere than after those of the nondominant hemisphere. Two possible explanations come to mind to explain the greater impairment in patients with left-hemisphere lesions. Gainotti (1972) and Heilman and co-workers (1975) noted the tendency for right-hemisphere-damaged patients to have decreased emotional responses or even a euphoric-like state, whereas patients with left-hemisphere lesions tend to be depressed. This may also explain a report by Cole and Patawaran *(personal communication)* of 3 patients who, following a right-hemisphere stroke, developed sexual hallucinations, sexual delusions, and a tendency to use obscene language quite inappropriately. Similar anecdotes were reported by Weinstein (1974) and Weinstein and Kahn (1955) who denied any relationship between this type of behavior and lesion side, although several of their disinhibited patients had left hemiplegia.

Another possible explanation for the greater loss of libido following left-hemisphere lesions is related to their effect on language. Malone (1975) distributed a questionnaire about sexual relationships to the wives of male aphasics under treatment at the VA Hospital in Houston. Her goal was to determine whether or not, from the wives' point of view, changes existed in sexual relationships after stroke in that aphasic population. Malone also wanted to know if these changes were of concern to the wives. Sixteen wives satisfactorily completed the questionnaire. The sexual relationship was "less satisfactory than before the stroke" in 13 of the 16 cases (81%). In 12 cases (75%), the frequency of sexual intercourse was decreased, whereas 2 wives reported greater frequency of intercourse. Of the 16 wives, 8 stated that they were "unconcerned" about these changes, 4 were "slightly concerned," and 4 were "greatly concerned."

Since no normal controls and no patients with stroke but without aphasia were included in the study, the specific importance of language impairment cannot be assessed. Comparison of Malone's results with those of Kalliomaki and co-workers (1961) is difficult because Malone did not directly investigate libido and did not include controls with no language impairment. This study, therefore, does not allow any conclusion regarding the relationship between language disorders and the significantly greater number of patients who suffered a decreased libido following left-hemisphere lesions. Concerning frequency of coitus, however, both studies come up with strikingly similar figures; that is, approximately three-fourths of male patients reported a decreased coital frequency. Another study by Wiig (1973) on sexual readjustment of aphasic patients allows a better understanding of the possible relationship between language disorders and sexual impairment. Wiig noted that, in her group, "Aphasics with relatively good auditory comprehension and nonverbal communication ability exhibited the least problems in sexual adjustment, irrespective of expressive language ability." On the other hand, patients with disorders of comprehension tended to show greater difficulties in sexual adjustment. It is known that aphasics with disorders of auditory comprehension also have impaired comprehension of nonverbal visual material such as symbolic gestures (Gainotti and Lemmo, 1976) and nonverbally expressed emotions (Gainotti, 1972). Wiig and colleagues (1973) think, therefore, that their patients' inability to interpret "body language" may have been the cause of the sexual anxieties, rejection, and frustrations as well as the social and sexual conflicts reported by patients with poor comprehension. One should also keep in mind that many patients with poor comprehension have temporal lobe lesions, but Wiig's data do not allow any speculation on the possible concomitant role of this anatomical factor.

In conclusion, it appears from these very few systematic studies that strokes (and presumably other cerebral lesions) may impair both libido and coital frequency. Better knowledge of the specific role of motor impairment and affective and cognitive factors would be very important for the purpose of prognosis and therapy.

Other Lesions

Other types of lesions have been said to be accompanied by depressed sexual functions. For example, it has been stated that patients with head injuries (Stier, 1938), particularly boxers (Mawdsley and Ferguson, 1963), tend to be hyposexual. Electroconvulsive therapy is also followed, at times, by impaired sexual behavior (Weinstein et al., 1952). Hierons and Saunders (1966) stated (without supporting data) that "degenerative disorders such as Alzheimer's disease may produce impotence." To date no systematic study has investigated the relationship between dementia and sexual behavior. Epilepsy has been discussed in a previous section. Counseling of both patient and spouse is an essential step in the management of patients with strokes and other hemispheric lesions.

One factor that may limit patients' ability to resume sexual activity after a stroke or myocardial infarction is perhaps the fear that intercourse may precipitate a new vascular complication. Certainly vascular accidents (particularly rupture of aneurysms and arteriovenous malformations) have been known to occur during intercourse (Viewpoints, 1969), but this does not seem to be a frequent occurrence. Ueno (1963) studied 5,559 autopsy cases of sudden deaths and found only 34 cases (0.61%) in which death was apparently related to sexual activities. Of the 28 males autopsied, the majority (18 patients) dies of cardiac causes, whereas the majority of the females (4 out of 6) died of cerebral hemorrhage.

DRUGS AFFECTING SEXUAL BEHAVIOR

Table 4 summarizes the effect on sexual functions of some commonly used drugs. As can be noted from this table, almost nothing is known about the effect of drugs on female sexual functioning.

TABLE 4. *Effect of some commonly used drugs on sexual behavior*[a]

	Males			Females
	Libido	Erection	Ejacul.	
Antihypertensive drugs				
Clonidine	N	−	N	?
Ganglionic blocking agents	N	−	−	?
Rauwolfia serpentina	−	N	−	?
Guanethidine	N	N	−	?
Methyldopa	−	N	−	?
Alpha-adrenergic blocking agents	N	N	−	?
Drugs used in psychiatry				
Antidepressants				
Anti-MAO	N	N	−	?
Tricyclic antidepressants	N	−	N	?
Lithium	N	N	N	?
Antipsychotic	N or −	N	−	?
Antianxiety drugs	?N	N	−	?
Drugs for Parkinson's disease				
Cholinergic blocking agents	N	−	−	?
Adrenergic drugs	?+	N	N	?
Anticonvulsant agents	N	N	N	?N
Alcohol	N or +	−	N	?−

[a]Legend: N = no change; + = increased; − = decreased; ? = no adequate information.

Antihypertensive Drugs

Clonidine (Catapres)

This is an antihypertensive drug with a complex mode of action (Yeh et al., 1971), in that it reduces sympathetic activity by a central action, and it also reduces the vascular effects of both vasoconstrictors and vasodilators. The drug induces dryness of the mouth, urinary retention, and difficulties with erection in 10 to 20% of males in chronic therapy (Nickerson and Collier, 1975). This suggests that the drug may interfere with parasympathetic function, although it is generally considered an adrenergic partial antagonist.

Ganglionic Blocking Agents

Drugs, such as tetraethylammonium and hexamethonium had been known for many years, but were not thoroughly investigated until after World War II (Acheson and Moe, 1946); they were introduced into clinical practice a few years later. These agents block nicotinic cholinergic receptors in both sympathetic and parasympathetic autonomic ganglia. Paton (1954) has given a vivid account of the hexamethonium man:

> He is a pink complexioned person, except when he has stood in a queue for a long time, when he may get pale and faint. His handshake is warm and dry. He is a placid and relaxed companion, for instance, he may laugh, but he can't cry because the tears cannot come. Your rudest story will not make him blush, and the most unpleasant circumstances will fail to make him turn pale. His collars and socks stay very clear and sweet. He wears corsets and may, if you meet him out, be rather fidgety (Corsets to compress his splanchnic vascular pool, fidgety to keep the venous return going from his legs). He dislikes speaking much unless helped with something to moisten his dry mouth and throat. He is long-sighted and easily blinded by bright light. The redness of his eyeballs may suggest irregular habits and in fact his head is rather weak. But he always behaves like a gentleman and never belches nor hiccups. He tends to get cold and keeps well wrapped up. But his health is good; he does not have chillblains and those diseases of modern civilization, hypertension and peptic ulcer, pass him by. He is thin because his appetite is modest; he never feels hunger pains and his stomach never rumbles. He gets rather constipated so that his intake of liquid paraffin is high. As old age comes on, he will suffer from retention of urine and impotence, but frequency, precipitancy and strangury will not worry him. One is uncertain how he will end, but perhaps if he is not careful, by eating less and less and getting colder and colder, he will sink into a symptomless, hypoglycemic coma and die, as was proposed for the universe, a sort of entropy death.

Impotence occurs because the parasympathetic blockage interferes with erection and also because the sympathetic blockage interferes with the emission of semen. Because of their side effects, ganglionic blocking agents are no longer commonly used in current practice.

Rauwolfia Alkaloids

Reserpine and the other alkaloids present in *Rauwolfia serpentina* act primarily by causing a depletion of catecholamines and serotonin in the central and peripheral nervous system. This depletion is primarily the result of a blockage of vesicle uptake of the previously released amine, which subsequently is metabolized. The blockage is irreversible, and new vesicles must be synthesized (Iversen, 1967); therefore, less norepinephrine is available as a neurotransmitter. The degree of sympathetic blockade may sometimes be of sufficient magnitude to interfere with semen emission. A very high incidence of depression is seen in patients treated with these drugs, and a decreased sex drive may also be a direct result of their action. Galactorrhea and extrapyramidal symptoms (tremor and rigidity) have also been observed. These complications rarely occur with the usual antihypertensive doses.

Guanethidine (Ismalin)

This drug has a complex pharmacological action. Experimental intravenous injection first produces a transient rise of blood pressure (tyramine-like effect), followed by interferences with conduction of nerve impulses and a defective catecholamine release (bretylium-like effect). Catecholamines in the nerve fibers are depleted (reserpine-like effect), and finally a block of neuronal catecholamine uptake occurs (cocaine-like effect) (Boura and Green, 1965). However, in contrast to the effects caused by reserpine, guanethidine does not cause sedation and depression, because it does not penetrate the blood-brain barrier. Orthostatic hypotension is frequently seen. The drug's effect on male sexual function is paradoxical; it does not interfere with sex drive, erection, and orgasm, but reduced emission and delay or failure of ejaculation occurs in as many as 60% of patients on large doses (Mills, 1975). This effect is not due to retrograde ejaculation but is probably secondary to absent contraction of the seminal vesicle, ampulla, and ductus deferens. On this basis, it has been suggested that guanethidine, and perhaps other drugs that reduce ejaculation might serve as reversible male contraceptives (Kedia and Markland, 1975).

Methyldopa (Aldomet)

Because of its low substrate specificity, dopamine beta-hydroxylase oxidizes almost any phenylethylamine to its corresponding phenylethanolamine (Cooper et al., 1978). Methyldopa is therefore taken up into synaptic vesicles and hydroxylated to alphamethylnorepinephrine. Since it is not as effective as norepinephrine, it functions as a false neurotransmitter and, as a result, decreases sympathetic activity. As is probably the case with many other drugs, the frequency of occurrence of sexual difficulties is related to dosage. At doses lower than 1.0 g per day, decreased libido is reported by 10 to 15% of patients of both sexes, with men also complaining of impotence. This percentage rises to 20 to 25% for doses from 1.0 to 1.5 g and reaches 50% for doses of 2 g or more (Kolodny, 1978). Reduced emission and difficulty with ejaculation are common problems. A decreased sex drive is also common, probably due to the drug's direct CNS action. Galactorrhea (due to prolactin release because dopamine action is decreased) has also been reported.

Alpha-Adrenergic Antagonists

Drugs such as phenoxybenzamine (Dibenzyline), phentolamine (Regitine), and tolazoline (Priscoline) block the effect of norepinephrine on blood vessels, unmasking the dilator (beta-adrenergic) effect of epinephrine (Weiner, 1980). As a result of this adrenergic blocking action, emission and ejaculation may be impaired, although sex drive, erection, and orgasm remain intact. Although used initially as antihypertensives, these drugs are of little value for that purpose and are used mainly in specific circumstances (e.g., for the diagnosis of pheochromocytoma) for short periods of time.

Management of Sexual Side Effects of Antihypertensive Medications

As can be seen from the preceding discussion, nearly all drugs and procedures (Allen and Adams, 1938) used for the treatment of hypertension may in one way or another interfere with sexual functions. A combination of agents leading to a lower dosage or discontinuation of the drugs best known for their side effects on sexual functions may minimize this problem (Oaks and Moyer, 1972). Howard (1973) advocates the specific combination of a diuretic, hydralazine, and propanolol [which, however, can also induce impotence, as noted by Zacharias (1976)] as one that keeps sexual side effects to a minimum. Of course this is possible only when more potent antihypertensives are not necessary. Many authors have commented on the low rate of compliance among patients on antihypertensive therapy (e.g., Sacket et al., 1975). The role drug side effects on sexual functioning play in low compliance to these drugs has not been studied but should be considered by all physicians who treat hypertensive patients (Murphy, 1978).

Drugs Used in Psychiatry

Antidepressants

Monoamine Oxidase Inhibitors

Monoamine oxidase (MAO) inhibitors were introduced into clinical practice as antidepressants after Zeller and colleagues (1952) found that the chemotherapeutic agent, iproniazid (which had been noted to have a mood-elevating effect in tubercular patients) was capable of inhibiting the enzyme MAO, which in turn increased the amount of available norepinephrine. Paradoxically, MAO inhibitors have been reported to delay emission and inhibit ejaculation, but the pharmacological basis of these effects is not clear. The MAO inhibitors have a potential use in hypertension, narcolepsy, and depression but are no longer widely used due to their toxicity.

Tricyclic Antidepressants

This class of drugs, which includes imipramine (Tofranil), amitriptyline (Elavil), and nortriptyline (Aventyl) blocks the transport system of the axonal membrane for reuptake of norepinephrine. This tends to potentiate sympathetic responses in addition to having a central cholinergic effect. This latter action is responsible for most of the side effects of these drugs. Sex drive is variously affected, sometimes being increased (perhaps in relation to patients' mood elevations), sometimes decreased. Failure of erection has been reported in some patients (Mills, 1975).

Lithium

Lithium has been shown to have some effectiveness in the treatment of affective psychosis, particularly in the manic phase of manic-depressive psychosis. Disturbed sexual functions (impaired erection) have occasionally been reported (Hollister, 1975). However, disturbed sexual function is common in such patients, and lithium can be regarded as having no major effect on sexual function.

Antipsychotic Drugs

The antipsychotic drugs are divided into phenothiazine [e.g., chlorpromazine (Thorazine), fluphernazine (Vesprin), and thioridazine (Mellaril)], thioxantone [e.g., chlorprothixene (Taractan)] and butyrophenone [haloperidol (Haldol)]. Although all these drugs have complex pharmacological actions, their primary characteristic seems to be a blockage of the effect of dopamine (Baldessarini, 1980). In addition, some antipsychotic drugs are weak cholinergic and alpha-adrenergic antagonists. Thioridazine in particular produces cholinergic blockage due to an atropine-like action on parasympathetic receptors. All these drugs have been reported to occasionally affect sexual behavior (Mills, 1975), particularly thioridazine (Kedia and Markland, 1975), which tends to interfere with ejaculation.

Antianxiety Drugs

Chlordiazepoxide (Librium), diazepam (Valium), oxazepam (Serax), and other benzodiazepines have infrequently been reported to affect sex drive, either increasing or decreasing it (Mills, 1975). The true incidence of this side effect is probably negligible.

Management of Sexual Side Effects of Drugs Used in Psychiatry

At the present time, we do not have a clear general understanding of the sexual side effects of drugs used in psychiatry. Research in this area has been limited by the failure of clinicians and researchers to establish preillness baseline levels of sexual interest and functioning. Admittedly, this is a difficult problem since the patients' recollection of their sexuality before their illness may well be colored by the illness itself; thus, the extremely depressed patient may recall his or her preillness interest or functioning in an exaggeratedly negative manner; and likewise, the manic patient is likely to have somewhat exaggerated recollections of interest and functioning. Research in the area is further complicated by the difficulty in separating the general effect of the medication on mood from the side effect of the medication on sexual functioning. The rules outlined for antihypertensive therapy side effects apply to these drugs, although one must keep in mind the added complication of distinguishing between sexual disorders which may be caused by the drugs and those caused by the disorder for which they are given. With respect to the individual patient, it is useful to try to establish as best as is possible what premorbid levels of sexual behavior and functioning were like. In the case of those patients with a consistent partner, information gathered from this collateral source can be extremely valuable in evaluating the effects of the drug on sexual functioning, as well as the effects of mood elevation or alteration on sexual functioning.

Narcotics and Analgesics

Most of our knowledge of the action of these drugs on sexual behavior derives from studies of their chronic use, and will be dealt with later (pp. 71–74).

Drugs Used in Parkinson's Disease

Cholinergic Blocking Agents

Atropine and synthetic anticholinergics all produce similar side effects such as dryness of the mouth, blurred vision, dizziness, and some urinary retention. Impaired erection and failure of ejaculation occur in some patients receiving high doses (Mills, 1975).

Adrenergic Drugs

Physicians involved in the treatment of male patients with Parkinson's disease are familiar with anecdotal reports of increased sex drive and sexual performance following levodopa and other adrenergic drugs. Rats with increased brain dopamine or decreased serotonin concentration tend to exhibit increased sexual activity (Gessa and Tagliamonte, 1975). One systematic study of sexual behavior during levodopa treatment in humans has shown that there tends, indeed, to be a slight improvement in sexual behavior, characterized by increased libido and greater coital frequency (Bowers and Van Woert, 1972). However, it is doubtful that this is due to a specific effect of the drug, and it is usually thought that whatever effect occurs is the result of improved motor activity and affect and to a consequent removal of sexual inhibition.

Anticonvulsant Agents

It is usually considered that anticonvulsant agents per se do not directly affect sexual behavior. Prolonged use of phenobarbital has been said to occasionally produce lack of libido and potency (Alpers and Mancall, 1971). This is probably a nonspecific effect due to CNS depression.

Sex Hormones

A detailed discussion of the effect of sex hormones on sexual function is not within the scope of this book. (See Martin et al., 1977; Adams et al., 1978; Rose, 1978; Kolodny et al., 1979 for recent reviews and points of view.) Testosterone and estrogen have been used in a variety of sexual impairments, but most authors agree that the use of these drugs to treat sexual inadequacy should be strictly limited to conditions in which hormone deficiencies are clearly documented. Some reports that sex hormones may be useful in the treatment of patients with spinal cord injuries (Cooper and Hoen, 1952) and diabetes (Schoffling et al., 1963), have remained isolated and unconfirmed.

Alcohol

Shakespeare's Porter (*Macbeth* Act II, Scene III) correctly observed that alcohol "provokes the desire, but takes away the performance." The paradoxical effect of acute doses of alcohol on sexual behavior has been known for many centuries. Chronic use of alcohol may seriously interfere with sexuality. Masters and Johnson (1966) and Kaplan (1974) all implicate heavy drinking as a major cause of decreased sexual responsivity. Lemere and Smith (1973) state that at least 8% of their alcoholic male patients who become abstinent complained of impotence, and in approximately 50% of these patients the effect persisted after years of sobriety. Chronic alcoholism is known to induce feminization, and on this basis, some authors (Van Thiel and Lester, 1974) have emphasized hormonal factors as being responsible for the sexual difficulties of these patients. Lemere and Smith (1973) noted, however, that sex drive was strong in all their patients. Since testosterone did not improve functioning in their male alcoholics, these authors concluded that impotence in alcoholics is due neither to hormonal nor to psychological factors but rather is secondary to autonomic neuropathy. Classical experiments in animals (Gantt, 1952) and more recent work in humans (Appenzeller and Richardson, 1966) seem to lend some support to the latter theory. It is possible that impotence with alcohol use is actually due to a combination of disorders of ANS and of CNS activity, and hormonal and psychogenic factors (Labby, 1975).

Experimental investigation of the relationship between alcohol consumption and objective measures of sexual arousal represents a relatively recent phenomenon. Using penile tumescence measurement during exposure to erotic stimuli, Farkas and Rosen (1976), Briddell and Wilson (1976), and Rubin and Henson (1976) all studied nonalcoholic young males and found essentially the same effect: decreasing penile tumescence with increasing alcohol consumption, often despite the subject's expectations and the subjective reports to the contrary.

As is the case for most potential sources of impaired sexual functions, information on the effect of alcohol on women is quite scarce. As stated by Carpenter and Armenti (1971), "Most experts comment on human sexual behavior and alcohol as though only males drink and have sexual interests." Few, if any, of Lemere and Smith's (1973) female patients complained of sexual inadequacy as a result of drinking. It is not clear, however, whether systematic inquiry regarding alterations in the sexual functioning was made of the female patients who, in general, are less likely to voice specific complaints. Lemere and Smith's findings contrast sharply with Kinsey's (1966) report that 72% of the 46 female alcoholics studied intensively by him were labeled as "frigid." Massot and co-workers (1957), Curran (1937), and Levine (1955) have all suggested that alcoholic women tend to be disinterested in sex, generally, and more so during acute intoxication. Wilson and Lawson (1976) studied the effect of alcoholic beverages on 16 female college students who were "moderate social drinkers and exclusively heterosexual." Subjects viewed a control film and an erotic film; their "erotic arousal" was measured by changes in their vaginal pressure pulse and blood volume monitored with a photoplethysmograph (Sinthak and Geer, 1975). Heart rate was also recorded. Arousal in response to the erotic film was significantly greater than during the control film. There was, however, an inverse correlation between the level of alcoholic consumption and physiologic arousal. If one were to assume that change in vaginal plethysmography is an adequate equivalent of sexual arousal, it would appear that the "Porter's effect," the increased libido produced by alcohol in Shakespeare's (and popular) belief, did not apply to women in this particular experiment.

Psychoactive Drugs

The number of illicit psychoactive drugs in current use is quite high; consequently, so is the number of anecdotal reports linking them to change in sexuality. Data are available on only a handful of them. A few comments apply to practically all illicit drugs: Most of them are used in the hope of achieving an increase in sex drive, sexual performance, and sexual pleasure. Even in the best controlled studies it is quite difficult to differentiate relatively nonspecific effects such as removal of behavioral inhibition or CNS depression from any specific action on the mechanisms related to sexual functions. Furthermore, it is difficult to separate the actual effects of these drugs from the expectation that they will have a positive effect on sexual functioning, since only a double-blind control study could permit the conclusion that it is the drug which impacts on sexual interest or functioning and, to date, no researcher has been able to undertake such a study using illicit drugs. Perusal of reports on the effects of practically all drugs leads to the conclusion that any improvement in sexual functioning is at best transient, and that most if not all of these drugs eventually lead to decreased sexual performance (Hollister, 1975).

Cannabis

This substance has been used for many years on the assumption that it enhances sexual behavior. Many of the actions of marijuana act as a stimulant and a sedative in the same manner as alcohol, and this may account for enhanced sex with small doses. At higher doses, however, CNS depression predominates and reverses this effect. Hollister (1975) quotes the 1894 report of the Indian Hemp Drug Commission that states that the hemp drugs have "no aphrodisiac power whatever; and, as a matter of fact, they are used by ascetics in this country with the ostensible object of destroying sexual appetite." A recent study (Kolodny et al., 1974) has claimed that chronic marijuana use (4 days a week for a minimum of 6 months) was associated with decreased plasma testosterone levels in young males. Of the 17 subjects studied, 6 had oligospermia, and 2 were impotent. This claim, however, was not confirmed by another study (Mendelson et al., 1974).

Natural Opiates and Synthetic Derivatives

Chronic opiate use is perhaps best documented as producing an almost universal impairment of sexual life, even though initial use may be accompanied by enhancement of sexual pleasure (De Leon and Wexler, 1973). Impairment of sexual functions seems to be particularly marked in methadone maintenance (Cicero, et al. 1975). Sexual impairment may, in part, be attributed to CNS depression, to hormonal factors [i.e., decrease in testosterone levels (Mendelson et al., 1975)], and, in the case of methadone, to direct alpha-adrenergic blocking action (Cicero et al., 1975). Sperm motility has also been found to be decreased during methadone use and, to a lesser degree, in heroin users.

Amphetamines

These drugs have a highly variable effect on sexual behavior. Ellinwood (1967) and Ellinwood and Rockwell (1975) have reported that 20% of amphetamine users experienced an increase in sexual activity. Others (Gossup et al., 1974) have found that amphetamine in conventional doses produced essentially no sexual change in men, but a definite impairment (decreased sexual drive) in women. Here again, chronic use of amphetamine tends to be associated with impaired sexual performance, both because of biogenic amine depletion and because the drug becomes a substitute for sex (Hollister, 1975).

Cocaine

Cocaine addicts describe euphoric effects of cocaine in terms practically identical to those used by amphetamine addicts (Jaffe, 1980). Cocaine in small doses has been observed to delay ejaculation. Again, chronic use tends to reduce sexual drive and cocaine becomes a substitute for sex.

Methaqualone (Quaalude)

This substance was synthesized in 1951 as a possible antimalaria agent; soon its hypnotic effect was noticed and it became marketed as a sedative-hypnotic. In the late 1960s, the rumor of its supposed aphrodisiac qualities spread widely and led to its abuse. (See Inaba et al., 1973; Pascarelli, 1973 for a review.) As noted by Hollister (1975), no one who took the drug as a prescriptive sedative-hypnotic has ever noticed such effects; claims for its special sexual properties are probably simply related to cerebral disinhibition.

Phencyclidine (PCP, "Angel Dust")

This substance is becoming one of the major drugs of abuse, second to marijuana. It deserves special attention because of the episodic unpredictable nature of the psychotic episodes it brings about (which, after a single dose, last for up to 6 to 8 weeks interspersed with nonpsychotic periods of behavior). Preoccupation with both sexual and religious thought is a major factor in the use of this drug. Sexual dysfunction and psychotic behavior are probably of both CNS and psychological origin (e.g., Allen and Young, 1978).

Treatment

Obviously, treatment of sexual side effects of drug abuse consists of the treatment of the addiction itself. This topic has been recently reviewed by Jaffe (1980). In the case of heroin addiction, it has been claimed that methadone maintenance improves sexual function (Cushman and Dole, 1973); however, as discussed previously (Cicero et al., 1975) methadone itself may produce sexual disorders.

Effect of Drugs on Female Sexual Behavior

With few exceptions (e.g., Adams et al., 1978; Rose, 1978), our knowledge of the effect of drugs of any type on female sexual behavior is extremely scanty. It is not possible at this point to state whether this is due to the fact that sexual functions of females are less readily affected by drugs than those of males or to lack of interest on the part of researchers, or to greater difficulties in establishing objective research criteria in the field of female sexuality (Rose, 1978).

AGING

Interest in the neurology and psychology of aging has risen considerably in the recent past. Several years ago Critchley (1959) proposed a list of neurological signs of "normal" aged persons that has remained classic. They include:

1. *Pupillary changes.* These consist of a tendency toward miosis and a sluggishness in reaction to light and accommodation that may reach complete unreactivity. These changes are due to structural changes of the muscle responsible for pupillary movement (sphincter pupillae).

2. *Ocular movements.* A decrease in upward gaze and, to a lesser extent in convergence movements is frequently observed.

3. *Arcus Senilis.* This consists of a crescentic strip of cloudiness that appears first in the lower and later in the upper part of the eyelid and often ends up forming a ring. This is the result of lipoid infiltration of tissues and may be correlated with hypercholesterolenemia.

4. *Muscular wasting.* This is frequently observed especially in the hands and is due to a decrease in number and in bulk of the individual muscle fibers.

5. *Tremor.* A fine tremor is similar to "essential" tremor and is commonly found in old age (tremor senilis). The pathological basis of this condition is not clear.

6. *Sensory examination.* A raise in threshold for sensory stimuli is frequently observed. This is true for light touch, pain and, above all, vibration sense. A decrease in blood supply to the white matter of the spinal cord has been advocated as a possible explanation of these findings but has not been proven so far. Special senses are also commonly affected leading to presbyopia, presbyacusis, and presbyageusia, i.e., impairment of eyesight, hearing, and taste, respectively.

7. *Reflexes.* A decrease in deep tendon reflex response is frequently found particularly affecting the ankle jerk and, to a lesser extent, the reflexes of the upper limbs. The abdominal, plantar, and cremasteric reflexes are also difficult to obtain. These decreases in reflex response do not necessarily reflect changes in the nervous system but may be due to changes in the tendons, ligaments, and perhaps muscles.

8. *Posture and gait.* Old persons often have postural and gait changes resembling those seen in Parkinson's disease. These consist of an attitude of "general flexion" and a shuffling gait accompanied at times by rigidity and paucity of facial expression (amimia). These findings may reflect changes in the extrapyramidal system. In fact it has been postulated that Parkinson's disease and the normal aging process may share a deficiency in the synthesis of catecholamines (McGeer, 1978).

9. *Changes in mental status.* It is popularly considered normal for an older person to have a decrease in intellectual abilities and the words senile and senility are often used, somehow euphemistically to characterize these changes. Recent research has cast doubt on the validity of the concept and the reader is referred to recent publications (e.g., Birren and Schaie, 1977).

As far as sexuality is concerned it is a common observation that there is normally a gradual reduction with age in the frequency of copulation and all types of sexual behavior (Bromley, 1974). It is also true, however, that this is not a necessary concomitant of aging; sexual behavior between suitable partners sometimes occurs until quite late in life (Pfeiffer, 1974), and the often observed decrease is due in a sizable part to such nonspecific conditions as an intercurrent medical or neurological disease, a psychiatric disorder, particularly depression (Butler, 1975) and social and environmental pressure (Glover, 1975). Hormonal changes are also known to occur in both males and females. As can be seen, the majority of changes thought to produce a decrease in sexual functions in the elderly are nonspecific rather than strictly neurological.

REFERENCES

Acheson GH, Moe GK: The action of tetraethylammonium ion on the mammalian circulation. *J Pharmacol Exp Ther* 87:220–236, 1946.

Adams DB, Gold AR, Burt AD: Rise in female-initiated sexual activity at ovulation and its suppression by oral contraceptives. *N Engl J Med* 299:1145–1150, 1978.

Adams RD, Victor M: *Principles of Neurology*. New York:McGraw Hill, 2nd edition, 1981.

Allen EV, Adams WA: Physiologic effects of extensive sympathectomy in hypertension: *Ann Int Med* II:2151–2171, 1938.

Allen RM, Young SJ: Phencyclidine induced psychosis. *Am J Psychiatry* 135:1081–1084, 1978.

Alpers BH, Mancall EL: *Clinical Neurology*. Philadelphia: Davis, 1971.

Anastasopoulos C: Hypersexualität, Wesenänderung, Schlafstörungen und Demenz bei einem Tumor des rechten Schafenlappen. *Psychiatr Neurol* 136:85–103, 1958.

Appenzeller O: *The Autonomic Nervous System*. Amsterdam: North Holland Publishing Co., 1976.

Appenzeller O, Richardson EP: The sympathetic chain in patients with diabetic and alcoholic polyneuropathy. *Neurology* 16:1205–1209, 1966.

Ayd FG, Blackwell B: *Discoveries in Biological Psychiatry*. Philadelphia: JB Lippincott, 1970.

Bailey GL: The sick kidney and sex. *N Engl J Med* 296:1288–1289, 1977.

Baldessarini RJ: Drugs and the treatment of psychiatric disorders. In: *Goodman and Gilman's The Pharmacological Basis of Therapeutics.* Goodman LS, Gilman A (Eds) Sixth Edition, New York: Macmillan, 1980, Chap 19, 391–447.

Bancaud J, Favel P, Bonis A, et al: Manifestations sexuelles paroxystiques et épilepsie temporale. *Rev Neurol* 123:217–230, 1970.

Barbeau A, Mars H, Gillo-Joffrey L: Adverse clinical side-effects of Levodopa therapy. In: *Recent Advances in Parkinson's Disease.* McDowell FH and Markham CH (Eds) Philadelphia: Davis, 1971.

Bard P: Central nervous mechanisms for emotional behavior patterns in animals. *Res Publ Assoc Res Nerv Ment Dis* 19:190–218, 1939.

Bardach JL: Sexuality in the disabled:some current work clinical, training, and research aspects. *Bull NY Acad Med* 54:510–516, 1978.

Barns RJ, Downey JA, Fremin DB, et al: Autonomic dysfunction with orthostatic hypotension. *Aust NZ J Med* 1:15–21, 1971.

Bauer HG: Endocrine and Metabolic conditions related to pathology in the hypothalamus: A review. *J Nerv Ment Dis* 128:323–338, 1959.

Beach FA: Effects of cortical lesions upon the copulatory behavior of male rats. *J Comp Psychol* 29:193–244, 1940.

Bear DM, Fedio P: Quantitative analysis of interictal behavior in temporal lobe epilepsy. *Arch Neurol* 34:456–467, 1977.

Becker LE, Mitchell AD: Priapism. *Surg Clin North Am* 45:1522–1534, 1965.

Berry PR: Neurological complications of haemophilia. *NZ Med J* 81:427–428, 1975.

Birren JE, Schaie KW (Eds): *Handbook of the Psychology of Aging.* New York: Van Nostrand and Reinhold Co., 1977.

Blumer D: Hypersexual episodes in temporal lobe epilepsy. *Am J Psychiatry* 126:1099–1106, 1970.

Blumer D, Benson DF: Personality changes with frontal and temporal lobe lesions. In: *Psychiatric Aspects of Neurologic Disease.* Benson DF and Blumer D (Eds) New York: Grune and Stratton, 1975.

Blumer D, Walker AE: Sexual behavior in temporal lobe epilepsy. *Arch Neurol,* 16:7–43. 1967.

Blumer D, Walker AE: The neural basis of sexual behavior. In: *Psychiatric Aspects of Neurologic Disease.* Benson DF and Blumer D (Eds) New York: Grune and Stratton, 1975, Chap 11, 199–217.

Bonica JJ: Autonomic innervation of the viscera in relation to nerve block. *Anesthesiology* 29:793–813, 1968.

Bors E, Canan AE: *Neurological Urology.* Basel: Karger, 1971.

Bors E, Turner RD: History and physical examination in neurologic urology. In: *The Neurogenic Bladder*. Boyarsky S (Ed) Baltimore: Williams & Wilkins, 1967, 64–74.

Boura ALA, Green AF: Adrenergic neurons blocking agents. *Annu Rev Pharmacol* 5:183–212, 1965.

Bowers MB, Van Woert MH: Sexual behavior during L Dopa treatment of Parkinson's disease. *Med Asp Hum Sex* 1:88–98, 1972.

Bradbury S, Eggleston C: Postural hypotension. A report of 3 cases. *Am Heart J* 1:72–86, 1925.

Bradbury S, Eggleston C: Postural hypotension. Autopsy on a case. *Am Heart J* 3:105–106, 1927.

Brain WR, Wilkinson M: *Cervical Spondylosis*. Philadelphia, Saunders, 1967.

Briddel DW, Wilson GT: Effects of alcohol and expectancy set on male sexual response. *J. Abnorm Psychol* 85:225–234, 1976.

Brodal A: *Neurological Anatomy*. Third Edition. New York: Oxford University Press, 1981.

Bromley DB: *The Psychology of Human Aging*. London: Penguin, 2nd Edition, 1974.

Brooks MH: Effects of diabetes on female sexual response. *Med Asp Hum Sex* 11:63–64, 1977.

Butler RN: Psychiatry and the elderly: an overview. *Am J Psychiatry* 132:893–900, 1975.

Carpenter JA, Armenti NP: Some effect of ethanol on human sexual and aggressive behavior. In: *The Biology of Alcoholism*. Kissin B, Begleiter H (Eds) New York: Plenum, 1971, Vol. 2.

Cartlidge NEP: Autonomic function in multiple sclerosis. *Brain* 95:661–664, 1972.

Cicero TJ, Bell RD, Wiest WG, et al: Function of male sex organ in heroin and methadone users. *N Engl J Med* 292:882–886, 1975.

Cohen AS: Amyloidosis. In: *Principals of Internal Medicine*. Isselbacher KJ, Adams RD, Braunwald E, et al (Eds) New York: McGraw Hill, 1980, Chap 64, 338–341.

Cohen AS, Benson MD: Amyloid Neuropathy. In: *Peripheral Neuropathy*. Dyck PJ, Thomas PK, Lambert EH (Eds) Philadelphia: Saunders, 1975, Chap 53, 1067–1091.

Comarr AE: Sexual function among patients with spinal cord injury. *Urol Int* 25:134–168, 1970.

Comarr AE: Sexual function in spinal cord injury patients. Diagnosis and Therapy: *Urology* 1:1–18, 1975.

Cooper AJ: The causes and management of impotence. *Postgrad Med J* 48:548–552, 1972.

Cooper IS, Hoen TI: Metabolic disorders in paraplegics. *Neurology* 2:332–340, 1952.

Cooper JR, Bloom FE, Roth RH: *The Biochemical Basis of Neuropharmacology*, Third Edition. New York: Oxford University Press 1978.

Critchley M: Neurological changes in the aged. *J Chronic Dis* 3:459–477, 1959.

Cushman P, Dole V: Detoxification of rehabilitated maintained patients. *JAMA* 226:747–752, 1973.

Curran F: Personality studies in alcoholic women. *J Nerv Ment Dis* 86:645–667, 1937.

Currier RD, Little SC, Sness JF, et al: Sexual seizures. *Arch Neurol* 25:260–266, 1971.

Dahlberg CC, Jaffe J: *Stroke. A Doctor's Personal Story of His Recovery*. New York: Norton, 1977.

De Jong RN: *The Neurological Examination*. Fourth Edition. Hagerstown: Harper & Row, 1979.

De Leon C, Wexler HK: Heroin addiction: its relation to sexual behavior and sexual experience. *J. Abnorm Psychol* 81:36–38, 1973.

Dewhurst K, Oliver JE, McKnight AL: Sociopsychiatric consequences of Huntington's disease. *Br J Psychiatry* 116:255–258, 1977.

Dua S, MacLean PD: Localization for penile erection in medial frontal lobe. *Am J Physiol* 207:1425–1434, 1964.

Dyck PS, Thomas PK, Lambert EH (Eds): *Peripheral Neuropathy*. Philadelphia: Saunders, 1975.

Eisenberg M: Sex and disability: selected bibliography. *J Rehab Psychol* 25:59–113, 1978.

Eisenberg MC, Rastad LC: Development of a sex counseling and education program on a spinal cord injury service. *Arch Phys Med Rehab* 57:135–140, 1976.

Ellenberg M: Impotence in diabetes: the neurologic factor. *Ann Intern Med* 75:213–219, 1971.

Ellenberg M: Impotence in diabetes: the neurologic factor. In: *Handbook of Sex Therapy*. Lo Piccolo J, Lo Piccolo L (Eds) New York: Plenum Press, 1978, Chap 33, 421–432.

Ellinwood EH: Amphetamine psychosis: Description of the individuals and process. *J Nerv Ment Dis* 144:273–283, 1967.

Ellinwood EH, Rockwell WJ: Effect of drug use on sexual behavior. *Med Asp Hum Sex* 9:10–32, 1975.

Erickson T: Erotomania (nymphomania) as an expression of cortical and epileptiform discharge. *Arch Neurol Psychiatr* 53:226–231, 1945.

Ertekin C, Reel F: Bulbocavernosus reflex in normal men and in patients with neurogenic bladder and/or impotence. *J Neurol Sci* 28:1–15, 1976.

Evans TN: Sexually transmissible diseases. *Am J Obstet Gynecol* 125:116–133, 1976.

Ewing OJ, Campbell IW, Burt AA, et al: Vascular reflexes in diabetic autonomic neuropathy. *Lancet* 2:1353–1356, 1973.

Farkas GM, Rosen RC: Effect of alcohol on elicited male sexual response. *J Stud Alcohol* 37:265–272, 1976.

Fisher C, Gross J, Zuch J: Cycle of penile erection syndromes with dreaming (REM) sleep. *Arch Gen Psychiatry* 12:29–45, 1965.

Fisher C, Schiavi R, Lear H, et al: The assessment of nocturnal REM erection in the differential diagnosis of impotence. *J Sex Marital Ther* 1:277–289, 1975.

Ford AB, Orfiren AP: Sexual behavior and the chronically ill patient. *Med Asp Hum Sex* 8:10–30, 1976.

Frank E, Anderson C, Rubinstein D: Frequency of sexual dysfunction in "normal" couples. *N Engl J Med* 299:111–115, 1978.

Freeman W: Sexual behavior and fertility after frontal lobotomy. *Biol Psychiatry* 6:97–104, 1973.

Furlow WL: Evaluation of the impotent patient. In: *Clinical Neuro-urology*. Krame RJ, Sinoky MB (Eds) Boston: Little, Brown & Co., 1979, Chap 8, 135–158.

Gainotti G: Emotional behavior and hemispheric side of the lesion. *Cortex* 8:41–55, 1972.

Gainotti G, Lemmo MA: Comprehension of symbolic gestures in aphasia. *Brain Lang* 3:451–460, 1976.

Gantt WH: Effect of alcohol on the sexual reflexes of normal and neurotic male dogs. *Psychosom Med* 14:174–181, 1952.

Gastaut H, Collomb H: Etude du comportement sexuel chez les épileptiques psychomoteurs. *Ann Med Psychol* 2:657–696, 1954.

Gastaut H, Mileto G: Interpretation physiopathogénique des symptomes de la rage furieuse. *Rev Neurol (Paris)* 92:5–25, 1954.

Gautier-Smith PC: Atteinte des fonctions cérébrales et troubles du comportement sexuel. *Rev Neurol (Paris)* 136:311–319, 1980.

Gessa GL, Tagliamonte P: Role of grain mono-amines in male sexual behavior. *Life Sci* 14:425–436, 1976.

Glover BH: Problems of aging: sex in the aging. *Postgrad Med* 57:165–169, 1975.

Goddess ED, Wagner NN, Silverman DR: Poststroke sexual activity of CVA patients. *Med Asp Hum Sex* 13:16–30, 1979.

Golji H: Experience with penile prosthesis in spinal cord injury patients. *J Urol* 121:288–289, 1979.

Goller H, Paeslack V: Pregnancy damage and birth complications in the children of paraplegic women. *Paraplegia* 10:213–217, 1972.

Gossup MR, Stern R, Connell PH: Drug dependence and sexual dysfunction. *Br J Psychiatr* 124:431–434, 1974.

Graber B, Kline-Graber G: Female orgasm: role of pubococcygeus muscle. *J Clin Psychiatr* 40:348–351, 1979.

Green AW: Sexual activity and the postmyocardial infarction patient. *Am Heart J* 89:246–252, 1975.

Green JD, Clemente CD, deGroot J: Rhinencephalic lesions and behavior in cats. An analysis of the Klüver-Bucy syndrome with particular reference to normal and abnormal sexual behavior. *J Comp Neurol* 108:505–545, 1957.

Green LF, Kedalis PP, Weeks RE: Retrograde ejaculation of semen due to diabetic neuropathy: report of 4 cases. *Fertil Steril* 14:617–625, 1963.

Griffith ER, Trieschmann RB: Sexual functioning in women with spinal cord injury. *Arch Phys Med Rehabil* 56:18–21, 1975.

Guttman L: Clinical symptomatology of spinal cord lesions. In: *Handbook of Clinical Neurology.* Vinken PJ, Bruyn GW (Eds) Amsterdam: North Holland, 1969, Vol 2, 178–216.

Harlow JM: Recovery from the passage of an iron bar through the head. *Pub Mass Med Soc* 2:329–342, 1868.

Hartings MF, Pavlov MM, Davis FA: Group counseling of MS patients in a program of comprehensive care. *J Chronic Dis* 29:65–73, 1976.

Heath RG: Pleasure response of human subjects to direct stimulation of the brain: physiologic and psycho-dynamic considerations. In: *The Role of Pleasure in Behavior.* Heath RG (Ed) New York: Harper & Row, 1964, 219–243.

Heath RG: Modulation of emotion with a brain pacemaker. *J Nerv Ment Dis* 165:300–317, 1977.

Heath RG, Harper JW: Descending projection of the rostal septal region: an electrophysiological-histological study in the cat. *Exp Neurol* 50:536–560, 1976.

Heilman KM, Scholes R, Watson RT: Auditory affective agnosia. *J Neurol Neurosurg Psychiatry* 38:69–72, 1975.

Hierons R, Saunders M: Impotence in patients with temporal lobe lesions. *Lancet* 2:761–764, 1966.

Higgins GE: Sexual response in spinal cord injured adults: A review of the literature. *Arch Sex Behav* 8:173–196, 1979.

Himmelhoch JM, Detre T: The unicorn in the garden. *(Unpublished manuscript).*

Hoenig J, Hamilton C: Epilepsy and sexual orgasm. *Acta Psychiatr Neurol Scand* 35:448–457, 1960.

Holdsworth S: The pituitary-testicular axis in man with chronic renal failure. *N Engl J Med* 296:1245–1249, 1977.

Hollister LE: Drugs and sexual behavior in man. *Life Sci* 17:661–666, 1975.

Howard EJ: Sexual expenditure in patients with hypertensive disease. *Med Asp Hum Sex* 7:88–92, 1973.

Inaba DS, Gay GR, Newmeyer JA, et al.: Methaqualone abuse—Luding out. *JAMA* 224:1505–1509, 1973.

Ivers RR, Goldstein NP: Multiple sclerosis: a current appraisal of symptoms and signs. *Mayo Clin Proc* 38:457–466, 1963.

Iversen LL: *The Uptake and Storage of Noradrenaline in Sympathetic Nerves.* Cambridge: The University Press, 1967.

Jaffe, JH: Drug addiction and drug abuse. In: *Goodman and Gilman's The Pharmacological Basis of Therapeutics.* Goodman LS, Gilman A (Eds) Sixth Edition, New York: Macmillan, 1980, Chap 16, 535–584.

Johnson RH, Spalding JMK: *Disorders of the Autonomic Nervous System.* Philadelphia: Davis, 1974.

Jovanovic UJ: A new method of phallography (PLG). *Confin Neurol* 29:299–312, 1967.

Kahn RA: Functional capacity of the isolated human spinal cord. *Brain* 73:1–51, 1950.

Kalliomaki JL, Markannen TK, Mustonen VA: Sexual behavior after cerebral vascular accident. *Fertil Steril* 12:156–158, 1961.

Kaplan HS: *The New Sex Therapy: Active Treatment of Sexual Dysfunctions.* New York: Brunner/Mazel, 1974.

Karacan I: Clinical value of nocturnal erection in the prognosis and diagnosis of impotence. *Med Asp Hum Sex* 4:27–34, 1970.

Karacan I, Goodenough DR, Shapiro A, et al: Erection cycle during sleep in relation to dream anxiety. *Arch Gen Psychiatry* 15:183–189, 1966.

Karacan I, Salis PJ, Ware JC, et al: Nocturnal penile tumescence and diagnosis in diabetic impotence. *Am J Psychiatry* 135:191–192, 1978.

Kedia K, Markland L: The effect of pharmacological agents on ejaculation. *J Urol* 114:569–573, 1975.

King DW, Ajmone Marsan CA: Clinical features and ictal patterns in epileptic patients with EEG temporal lobe foci. *Ann Neurol* 2:138–147, 1977.

Kinsey BA: *The Female Alcoholic.* Springfield: Thomas, 1966.

Klüver H, Bucy PC: Preliminary analysis of functions of the temporal lobes in monkeys. *Arch Neurol Psychiatr* 42:979–1000, 1939.

Kolodny RC: Sexual dysfunction in diabetic females. *Diabetes* 20:557–559, 1971.

Kolodny, RC: Effects of alpha-methyldopa on male sexual function. *Sex Disability* 1:223–228, 1978.

Kolodny RC, Kahn CB, Goldstein HH, et al: Sexual dysfunction in diabetic men. *Diabetes* 23:306–309, 1974.

Kolodny RC, Masters WH, Johnson VE: *Textbook of Sexual Medicine.* Boston: Little, Brown and Co., 1979.

Kolodny RC, Masters WH, Kolodner RM, et al: Depression of plasma testosterone levels after chronic intensive marijuana use. *N Engl J Med* 290:872–874, 1974.

Labby DH: Sexual concomitants of disease and illness. *Postgrad Med* 58:103–111, 1975.

Lapides J: Neuromuscular vesical and ureteral dysfunction. In: *Urology.* Campbell MF, Harrisson JH (Eds) Philadelphia: Saunders, 1976.

Lemere F, Smith JW: Alcohol induced sexual impotence. *Am J Psychiatry* 130:212–213, 1973.

Leriche R, Morel A: The syndrome of thrombotic obliteration of the aortic bifurcation. *Ann Surg* 127:193–206, 1948.

Levine J: The sexual adjustment of alcoholics: a clinical study of a selected sample. *Q J Stud Alcohol* 16:675–680, 1955.

Levine SB: Marital sexual dysfunction. *Ann Intern Med* 84:448–453, 1976.

Lezak MD: Living with the characterologically altered brain injured patient. *J Clin Psychol* 39:512–598, 1978.

Lilius HG, Valtonen EJ, Wilkstrom J: Sexual problems in patients suffering from multiple sclerosis. *J Chronic Dis* 29:643–647, 1976.

Lisk R: Sexual behavior: hormonal control. In: *Neuroendocrinology.* Martini L, Ganong WF (Eds) New York: Academic Press, 1967, Vol 2, 197–239.

Lorenz K: *Studies in Animal and Human Behavior.* Cambridge: Harvard University Press, 1970.

Low PA, Walsh JC, Huang CY, et al: The sympathetic nervous system in diabetic neuropathy. A clinical and pathological study. *Brain* 98:341–356, 1975.

Lundberg PO: Sexual dysfunction in multiple sclerosis. *Sexual Disab* 1:218–222, 1978.

MacLean PD: New findings on brain function and sociosexual behavior. In: *Contemporary Sexual Behavior.* Zubin J, Money J (Eds) Baltimore: Johns Hopkins University Press, 1973, 53–74.

MacLean PD, Denniston RH, Dua S: Further studies on cerebral representation of penile erection: caudal thalamus, midbrain and pons. *J Neurophysiol* 26:273–293, 1963.

MacLean PD, Dua S, Denniston RH: Cerebral localization for scratching and seminal discharge. *Arch Neurol* 9:485–497, 1963.

MacLean PD, Ploog DW: Cerebral representation of penile erection. *J Neurophysiol* 25:29–55, 1962.

Malone PE: A preliminary investigation of changes in sexual relations following strokes. In: *Clinical Aphasiology*. Brookshire RH (Ed) Minneapolis: BRK Publishers, 1975.

Martin JB, Reichlin S, Brown GM: *Clinical Neuroendocrinology*. Philadelphia: Davis, 1977.

Martin MM: Diabetic neuropathy. A clinical study of 150 cases. *Brain* 76:594–624, 1953.

Massot, Hamel, Deliry: Alcoholisme féminin: Données statistiques et psycopathologiques. *J Med Lyon* 37:265–269, 1956.

Masters WH, Johnson VE: *Human Sexual Response*. Boston: Little, Brown & Co., 1966.

Masters WH, Johnson VE: *Human Sexual Inadequacy*. Boston: Little, Brown & Co., 1970.

Mawdsley C, Ferguson FR: Neurological disease in boxers. *Lancet* 2:799–801, 1963.

McAlpine D, Lumsden CE, Acheson ED: *Multiple Sclerosis. A Reappraisal*. Edinburgh: Livingstone, 2nd Edition, 1972.

McGeer EG: Aging and neurotransmitter metabolism in the human brain. In: *Alzheimer's Disease, Senile Dementia and Related Disorders*; *Aging, Volume 7*, Katzman R, Terry RD, Bick K (Eds) New York: Raven Press, 1978.

Mendelson JH, Kuehnle L, Ellingbo J, et al: Plasma testosterone levels before, during and after chronic marihuana smoking. *N Engl J Med* 291:1051–1055, 1974.

Mendelson JH, Mendelson JE, Patch VD: Plasma testosterone levels in heroin addiction during methadone maintenance. *J Pharmacol Exp Ther* 192:211–217, 1975.

Meyers R: Evidence of a locus of the neural mechanisms for libido and penile potency in the septo-fornico-hypothalamic region of the human brain. *Trans Am Neurol Assoc* 86:81–85, 1961.

Meyers R: Central neural counterparts of penile potency and libido in humans and subhuman mammals. *Cincinn J Med* 44:281–291, 1963.

Mills LC: Drug induced impotence. *Am Fam Physician* 12:104–106, 1975.

Mitchell W, Falconer MA, Hill D: Epilepsy with fetishism relieved by temporal lobectomy. *Lancet* 2:626–630, 1954.

Moniz E: Prefrontal leucotomy in the treatment of mental disorder. *Am J Psychiatry* 93:1379–1385, 1937.

Murphy RS: Compliance dilemma: Antihypertensive and sexual dysfunction. *Behav Med* 5:10–14, 1978.

Nathan P: *The Nervous System.* Philadelphia: Lippincott, 1969, 198.

Nickerson M, Collier J: Antihypertensive agents and the drug therapy of hypertension. In: *The Pharmacological Basis of Therapeutics.* Goodman LS, Gilman A (Eds) New York: Macmillan, 1975, Chap 33, 705–726.

Nordborg C, Kristenssen K, Olsson Y, et al.: Involvement of the autonomous nervous system in primary and secondary amyloidosis. *Acta Neurol Scand* 49:31–38, 1973.

Nottebohm F, Arnold AP: Sexual dimorphism in vocal control areas of the songbird brain. *Science* 194:213, 1976.

Nottebohm F, Nottebohm ME: Left hypoglossal dominance in the control of canary and white crowned sparrow song. *J Comp Physiol A: Sens Neural Behav Physiol* 108:171–192, 1976.

Oaks WW, Moyer JH: Sex and hypertension. *Med Asp Hum Sex* 6:128–137, 1972.

Olivecrona H: The surgery of pain. *Acta Neurol Scand [Suppl]* 46:268–280, 1947.

Orback J, Milner B, Rasmussen T: Learning and retention in monkeys after amygdala hippocampus resection. *Arch Neurol* 3:230–251, 1960.

Partridge M: *Prefrontal Leucotomy.* Springfield: Thomas, 1960.

Pascarelli EF: Methaqualone abuse: The quiet epidemic. *JAMA* 226:1512–1514, 1973.

Paton WDM: The principles of ganglionic block. In: *Scientific Basis of Medicine.* London: Athlone Press, Vol 2, 1954.

Penfield W, Rasmussen T: *The Cerebral Cortex of Man.* New York: Macmillan, 1950.

Pfeiffer E: Sexuality in the aging individual. *J Am Geriatr Soc* 22:481–484, 1974.

Piera JB: The establishment of a prognosis for genitosexual function in the paraplegic and tetraplegic males. *Paraplegia.* 10:271–278, 1973.

Pinderhughes CA, Grace EB, Reyner LJ, et al: Interrelationships between sexual functioning and medical conditions. *Med Asp Hum Sex* 6:52–76, 1972.

Poeck K, Pilleri G: Release of hypersexual behavior due to a lesion in the limbic system. *Acta Neurol Scand* 41:233–244, 1965.

Porter RW, Bors E: Neurogenic bladder in Parkinsonism. *J Neurosurg* 34:27–32, 1971.

Pratt HM, Yin B, West WL: Bulbar spinal poliomyelitis complicating pregnancy at term. *N Engl J Med* 258:130–131, 1958.

Raisman, F, Field, PM: Sexual dimorphism in the preoptic area of the rat. *Science* 173:731–733, 1971.

Renshaw DC: Sexual problems of stroke patients. *Med Asp Hum Sex* 9:68–74, 1975.

Renshaw DC: Impotence in diabetics. In: *Handbook of Sex Therapy*. Lo Piccolo J, Lo Piccolo L (Eds) New York: Plenum Press, 1978, Chap 34, 433–440.

Riddoch G: The reflex functions of the completely divided spinal cord in man, compared with those associated with less severe lesion. *Brain* 40:264–402, 1917.

Robinson BW, Mishkin M: Penile erection evoked from forebrain structures in *Maccaca mulatta*. *Arch Neurol* 19:184–198, 1968.

Rose RM: Psychoendocrinology in the menstrual cycle. *N Engl J Med* 299:1186–1187, 1978.

Rosenblum JA: Human sexuality and the cerebral cortex. *Dis Nerv Syst* 35:268–271, 1974.

Rossier AB, Raffieux M, Ziegler WH: Pregnancy and labor in high traumatic spinal cord lesions. *Paraplegia* 7:210–216, 1969.

Rubin A, Babbott D: Impotence and diabetes mellitus. *JAMA* 168:498–500, 1958.

Rubin HB, Henson DE: Effects of alcohol on male sexual responding. *Psychopharmacologia* 47:123–134, 1976.

Sabri S, Cotton LT: Sexual functions following aortoiliac reconstruction. *Lancet* 2:1218–1219, 1971.

Sacket DL, Gibson ES, Taylor DW, et al: Randomized clinical trial of strategies for imposing medication compliance in primary hypertension. *Lancet* 1:1205–1207, 1975.

Saunders M, Rawson M: Sexuality in male epileptics. *J Neurol Sci* 10:577–583, 1970.

Schoffling K, Fedalia K, Ditschuneit H: Disorders of sexual functions in male diabetics. *Diabetes* 12:519–527, 1963.

Sharpey-Shafer EP: Circulatory reflexes in chronic disease of the afferent nervous system. *J Physiol* 134:1–10, 1956.

Sherman FP: Impotence in patients with chronic renal failure on dialysis: Its frequency and etiology. *Fertil Steril* 26:221–223, 1975.

Shy GM, Drager GA: A neurological syndrome associated with orthostatic hypotension. *Arch Neurol* 2:511–527, 1960.

Simpson SL: Impotence. *Br Med J* 1:692–697, 1950.

Sinthak G, Geer JA: A vaginal plethysmograph system. *Psychophysiology* 12:113–115, 1975.

Sjöstrand NO: The adrenergic innervation of the vas deferens and the accessory male genital glands. *Acta Physiol Scand* 65: Suppl 257:1–82, 1965.

Small MP: Differential diagnosis of impotence. *Med Asp Hum Sex* 12:55–56, 1978.

Smith JW, Lemere F, Dunn RB: Impotence in alcoholism. *Northwest Med* 71:523–526, 1972.

Special Correspondent: The forgotten: A man with motor neuron disease. *Br Med J* 2:40–41, 1971.

Stauffer CL, Frank E, Leb DE, et al: A survey of patients and the spouses who dialyze them. Paper presented at the Renal Roundtable Conference, Seven Springs, PA, October, 1980.

Stier E: Disturbances of sexual functions through head trauma. *J Nerv Ment Dis* 88:714–715, 1938.

Talbot HS: Sexual function in paraplegia. *J Urol* 73:91–100, 1955.

Tarabulcy E: Sexual function in the normal and in paraplegia. *Paraplegia* 10:201–208, 1972.

Taylor DC: Sexual behavior and temporal lobe epilepsy. *Arch Neurol* 21:510–516, 1969.

Terzian H, Dalle Ore G: Syndrome of Klüver-Bucy reproduced in man by bilateral removal of the temporal lobes. *Neurology* 5:373–380, 1955.

Thomas JP, Shields R: Associated autonomic dysfunction and carcinoma of the pancreas. *Br Med J* 4:32, 1970.

Thomas PK, Lascelles RG: The pathology of diabetic neuropathy. *Q J Med* 35:489–509, 1966.

Trieschman RB: The psychological, social and vocational adjustment in spinal cord injury. Easter Seal Society for crippled children and adults. Final report RSA 13-P-59011/9-01, 1978, Chap 7, 111–128.

Ueno M: The so-called coition death. *Japn J Leg Med* 17:330–340, 1963.

Van Thiel DH, Lester R: Sex and alcohol. *N Engl J Med* 291:251–253, 1974.

Vas CJ: Sexual impotence and some autonomic disturbances in men with multiple sclerosis. *Acta Neurol Scand* 45:166–182, 1969.

Victor M, Adams RD, Collins GH: *The Wernicke-Korsakoff Syndrome. Philadelphia: Davis, 1971.*

Viewpoints: Sudden death during coitus–fact or fiction? *Med Asp Hum Sex* 3:22, 1969.

Wasserman MD, Pallack CP, Spillman AJ, et al.: The differential diagnosis of impotence. *JAMA* 243:2038–2042, 1980.

Weiner N: Drugs that inhibit adrenergic nerves and block receptors. In: *The Pharmacological Basis of Therapeutics*, Goodman LS and Gilman A (Eds) New York: Macmillan, 1976, Chap 9, 176–210.

Weinstein EA: Sexual disturbances after brain surgery. *Med Asp Hum Sex* 8:10–18, 1974.

Weinstein EA, Kahn RL: *Denial of Illness*. Springfield: Thomas, 1955.

Weinstein EA, Linn L, Kahn RL: Psychosis during electroshock therapy. *Am J Psychiatry* 109:22–26, 1952.

Weiss AJ, Diamond D: Sexual adjustment, identification, and attitudes of patients with myelopathy. *Arch Phys Med Rehab* 4:245–250, 1966.

Weiss HD: The physiology of human penile erection. *Ann Intern Med* 76:92–799, 1972.

Wiig EH: Counseling the adult aphasic for sexual readjustment. *Rehab Couns Bull* 17:110–119, 1973.

Wiig EH, Strauss EC, Garwood PJ: Aphasic perception and interpretation of nonverbally expressed emotions. Paper presented at ASHA Annual Meeting, Detroit, Mich., October, 1973.

Wilson GT, Lawson DM: Effects of alcohol on sexual arousal in women. *J Abnorm Psychol* 85:489–497, 1976.

Yeh BK, Nantel A, Goldberg LI: Antihypertensive effect of clonidine. *Arch Intern Med* 127:233–237, 1971.

Young RF, Asbury AK, Corbett JL, et al.: Pure pan-dysautonomia with recovery. Description and discussion of diagnostic criteria. *Brain* 98:613–636, 1975.

Zacharias FJ: Patient acceptability of propranolol and the occurrence of side effects. *Postgrad Med J* 52(Suppl. 4): 87–89, 1976.

Zeller EA, Barsky J, Fouts JR, et al.: Influence of isonicotinic acid hydrazin (INH) and I-isonicotinyl2-isopropylhydrazide (IIN) on bacterial and mammalian enzymes. *Experientia* 8:349–350, 1952.

Subject Index

Subject Index